The C Card And Me 2

How I beat Stage IV cancer (again and again)

By

Ali Gilmore

DEDICATION

Dedicated to my mom, Alice Gilmore, and the other fighters in my family who took up the sword before me; Jim Gilmore, James Reeve Gilmore, Joel Duker, Laurie Gilmore, Leila Rie Serikaku-Takagi, Lisa Gilmore-Bell, and Susan Kahn.

ACKNOWLEDGMENTS

🚲 🚲 🚲

To my family and friends from across the globe (and possibly some far off planets), I am here today and have had so many great adventures post diagnosis. They are in many ways, thanks to you. You all know who you are and to you I say, "I love you love you love you~" I am one of the luckiest people on the planet for having you in my life.

I also want to send my deepest gratitude to the nurses and doctors who fight right alongside me, especially Dr. Derek Helton, my Oncologist/Handler. When you said it would be "a long road," I had no idea just how feckn long, but I'm glad you and your amazing team are on it with me. Also, a special thank you to Eve Beutler, MFT, and Mary Hollander, RN/RMT, for providing their expert input on the coping and nutrition chapters.

Last, but not least, I'd like to send a warm and appreciative shout out to Cancer Angels of San Diego for the support they give to the many Stage IV cancer fighters in San Diego County, ensuring each has a roof over their head, the lights on, healthy food in their bellies, and a way to/from treatment, allowing them to stay focused on the fight. I hope that many more communities will be inspired to do what they do, and the much needed funding will find its way to this 501C3 charity, so they can continue to make a real difference in real people's lives. Learn more about them at: www.cancerangelsofsandiego.org.

PROLOGUE

🚲 🚲 🚲

If you're reading this you may be someone who is proactive, and wanting to know ahead of time how you should deal with cancer if/when it comes your way. Current statistics show that 1 in 2 Americans will face it in their lifetime, so smart move on your part. That, or chances are you recently found out you or someone you love has cancer. Your world is about to change big-time and you're looking for some answers and direction.

Hey, I get it believe you me. I was diagnosed with Stage IV cancer in September of 2010. Since then, I've undergone one surgery to remove the tumor in my colon and another surgery to implant a port in my chest. I have been through 40-something (and counting) cycles of chemo, and spattered throughout that time, I've had targeted radiation therapy/radio surgery to get the cancer cells that had spread to my left lung (and then later, my right lung). I know how you feel. I've been there, done that (and though a bit wobbly) am still standing.

This isn't my first time at the (book) fair either, and some people might wonder why I'm writing a second cancer survival guide. Didn't I cover it all in the first one? Yes and no. The key things you need to know are covered in the first book. The second book expands on some topics, offers updates to the stories in the first (which makes it kind of cool to read them side by side), and adds some new info I've gained over the past few years, along with some input and guidance from experts I've met along the way. The first guide was written from the perspective of someone who had 18 months of cancer experience. I was hyper-wired and ecstatic thinking it was the last I'd have to deal with cancer directly. I thought I was passing on the baton, so to speak. I was also a bit manic in my approach because I had a deadline that I couldn't shift. I was writing it all out for a good friend's mother who had just been diagnosed late stage as I was wrapping up (what I thought was) my cancer treatment plan. Debbie, aka Debalou, and her mom Karolyn were the ones who encouraged me to publish it. Karolyn passed on just before the launch date, but she's forever honored in these books and remembered by me as the catalyst for the creation of these cancer survival guides, and my goal of making people less afraid of cancer and better prepared to face it.

Some things bear repeating from one book to the other. Most importantly, to acknowledge the fact that you are loved. If someone gave you this book, it's because that person doesn't want you to worry (and possibly they wanted to be promoted to the top of the list of your ultra cool and brilliant friends by giving you the best book ever). They want you to stick around on this planet. If you bought this for yourself, then good for you. You are now promoted to the top of my list of ultra cool and brilliant people. You love yourself enough to want to kick this thing's ass and believe you me that is the best place to start.

I think most everyone wants to feel that in the end, they've made a contribution to this world. I want to be able to proclaim, "I made over a million people less afraid of cancer, and better prepared to face it." My BFF (best friend forever), Michelle, says it's my calling. I say it might just be my *rai·son d'ê·tre.*

I'm also told that the book makes more sense if you are clued in on my writing style before forging ahead, so here it goes: I write like I speak, which generally gives you the feeling that we're sitting in a comfortable room somewhere chilling and just talking about real stuff like real people do. Well, this real person doesn't care much for grammatical rules and regulations. This tends to irritate some scholars, but my dad has a doctorate in education and he made it through the book without feeling any great shame or embarrassment, so there you have it.

Since I don't speak like an English textbook (faaar from it) when I tend to elongate words in speaking, I do so in writing. I'm also not a fan of the exclamation point. To me (and my slightly autistic brain), it sounds like yelling (which I don't like). I like to use the tilde (~) instead. It seems more lyrical and that's how my voice comes across when I'm excited about something. If I really want to emphasize something I will do it in ALL CAPS. That said, I have taken into account my BFF's gentle (ish) hint that there's such a thing as, "too much of a good thing," so I will try to curb it all in this edition.

Since *The C Card and Me* was first published, I've received some great feedback from readers with more than a few saying they wished I'd gone more in-depth on certain subjects, which I get, but I also think it's important to keep a cancer survival guide brief, something you can read in one sitting and really soak in. The first book was under 70 pages, and I've vowed to do my best to keep this one under 100 pages, so in an effort to provide more depth without too many more pages, we've combined two chapters to make room for two more and put loads of more in-depth coverage of the subjects on the website.

Just go to: www.theccardandme.com, type keywords like; *blood work, pee* or *coping,* etc., into the search field and you'll find the depth you're looking for. It's also a good way to keep key information up to date because as we all know, the world keeps evolving after books go to print.

Oh, and yes, you should know I tend to swear. Sometimes a lot. A society-savvy friend of mine informed me that swearing is, "less offensive if you misspell it." So, there you go.

I also like to use the infamous "dot dot dot" whenever I pause for effect. Last, but not least, I am ever experiencing the joys of chemo brain, so even with the help of a highly skilled editor you may come across something that doesn't quite fit into a sentence or paragraph or even a chapter. Sorry, I know it's annoying. Just take is as a shining example of what lies ahead...

So, if all that doesn't drive you around the bend, then by all means, please proceed. If it does, then seriously? Helloooooooo…we're facing cancer fer fkssake~ The sky will not fall, nor our society crumble under the weight of some illiterate smartarse's refusal to follow grammatical rules.

I do want to make it very clear though, this book in no way means any disrespect to those who've fought and lost. Not every battle can be won and every life has its own timeline. No one (and I mean no one) can guarantee your outcome, but a big, no, huuuge part of it is up to you. I hope this guide will smooth the path you're on, and shed a little light on an otherwise darker chapter in the book of life.

Ok, here it is…my gift to you. Here's a little more in-depth heads-up/insider info that should bring some peace of mind as well as direction. Life offers few guarantees. We are born, we live, and then we go off into the great beyond. If you're not quite ready for the last one, then it's time to get ready for the fight of and for your life…

CHAPTER 1
SO YOU'VE GOT IT. NOW WHAT?

🚲 🚲 🚲

So, the doc broke the bad news to you (gently or not so gently), and your head is reeling. I so get where you are coming from, I swear. I got my bit of news on my birthday of all days. For some reason, I expected it to be a happy, let's celebrate, kind of follow-up appointment after my colon surgery, body scan and biopsy, so I made it for an hour before meeting up with friends for the so-called "celebration" at our local martini bar.

I think I drank four or five martinis that night. I didn't even like martinis all that much back then (I have since developed a taste for them, thanks to the mad skills of Chandler, Michael and the rest of the gang), but I love my friends and we were all looking forward to celebrating, so that's what we did. I laughed at the stories and jokes and smiled like a Cheshire cat. All the while the words, "Technically it's Stage IV," kept whirling around my brain like a buzz saw. Man oh man, how I wish someone had, in that moment, done a quiet slide under the table, "Psst…here's a guide that'll get you through it all. No worries. Now, go enjoy the party." How great would that have been?

So, what's next on your agenda? Ask questions. The very first question out of your mouth should be, "Can you fix it?" If you haven't asked already, then ask now. Make 'em look you in the eye, tell you straight up what the chances are, and what treatment options are available. I asked the day I found out. Dr. H., my Oncologist, looked me straight in the eye and said, "Yes, but it'll be a long road." I responded with, "So what's the drama about? If you can fix it, then let's get to it." At the time, of course, I had no idea how long that "long road" was going to be, but I don't have any regrets about my attitude toward it all from day one.

Ask about your treatment options. Chances are, you are sitting down with someone who is well versed at chemo and/or radiation treatments. These are not the only options out there, and you should review them all before deciding, but I will give you my take on it. I say, "Fight fire with fire, then nurture with nature." If cancer is caused by the genetic mutation of healthy cells, then it makes sense to fight fire with fire first. Chemo/radiation is undoubtedly proven quite effective at eradicating cancer. Of this, I am living proof.

Cancer treatments are constantly evolving, and it is good to know your options. The *nurture with nature* mantra is targeted at the fact that a compromised immune system is linked to cancer, so once the chemo is over, you're going to need to blast your body with organic foods, supplements and a healthy lifestyle to restore what was depleted, and detox the residual chemicals from your body. In other words, blast those feckers out of your body, then rebuild.

You think that's BS? Then I've got two words for you; Steve Jobs. With all his positive mentality and money (both of which he had loads of), he opted the *nature* only method, and refused chemo/radiation. Look, there are over 100 different kinds of cancer and no two bodies alike so, of course, there is no patent answer to beating cancer (and don't you dare trust anyone who tells you there is), but they don't just throw any ole cancer drug at you. They run genetic testing to see which drug has responded best, based on your genetic markers. This method has made great strides in effectiveness of treatment. If I were diagnosed at Stage 1, maybe I would've been open to trying a more "natural" method of attack, but then again, I know a guy from Seattle who was recently diagnosed Stage 1. He went through just a few cycles, then he was in remission already. Three months out of your life for treatment is a cake walk compared to 4+ years and 40+ cycles, trust me.

Whatever treatment you decide, just be sure your eyes are wide open, you feel confident in it and those who are administering it. Then, ask for a list of side-effects. This is *muy importante*. I'll explain further about that in the "Bigger Boat" chapter. For now, focus on asking questions...

QUESTIONS TO ASK YOUR ONCOLOGIST

☐ Can you fix it? If you don't like the answer get a second and third opinion.

☐ What treatment options are available to me now?

☐ How long will treatment take, from start to finish? This is very important. I wasn't clear on this answer and it cost me a lot of time, money and stress in the end, so be prepared.

☐ What are the potential side effects?

☐ How long before the side effects kick in and how long will they last?

☐ What supplements should I be/not be taking and when?

☐ Is it safe to take antioxidants during or in-between chemo cycles?

☐ Why me? Why this particular cancer? They won't have a definitive answer, but you know you want to ask, so go on.

3

I can tell you I scratched my head quite a bit over, "How the fek could I get colon cancer when no one else in my family had it?" Cancer, yes. There are plenty of cases of that, but not colon cancer. That is, until my cousin recently discovered through her family tree hunt that my grandfather on my mother's side died of colon cancer. People weren't that big on talking about it 20 or more years ago, so just because you don't know of a history of any particular cancer in your family doesn't mean it isn't there...

Once you know your treatment plan, find out what your insurance company covers. You can't change what they cover, but you can be better prepared to open that bill when it comes. At one point during treatment, I opened a bill for $16,000. I think my heart actually stopped for a few seconds...then I sat down and went over in my head. I called the insurance company and found out someone had "accidentally flipped the numbers," so the huge amount was what the insurance company disallowed and the bill suddenly went from heart attack to relatively manageable...

QUESTIONS TO ASK YOUR INSURANCE COMPANY

☐ Inpatient (if surgery is part of the treatment plan).

☐ Outpatient (Port implants are considered outpatient surgery).

☐ Targeted Radiation Therapy (if it's part of the treatment plan).

☐ Home med equipment (if you have to use a portable chemo unit).

☐ Office visits (specialist and regular).

☐ CT and PET scans (you'll get these regularly).

☐ Is there just one cancer center in their network? It's always good to have choices.

☐ What about fertility treatments? If you're still fertile and want kids, you need to look at your options like freezing your stuff before chemo starts. Chemo doesn't just kill cancer cells. In most cases it will cause infertility in both sexes and early menopause in women, so be prepared.

What if you don't have insurance? It can be harder, but not impossible. Contact your state disability office, tell them your situation and ask what your options are. Of the dozens of people I've spoken to at that office, only one was unsympathetic, but he sounded like a miserable git with no love for life or people, so I let him and his crappy outlook roll right off my shoulders. In most cases, you will find people to be sympathetic and eager to help, but times are changing. Having cancer isn't as rare or devastating thing anymore, and after four years of it, people are as sick of my cancer as am I. It's nice when people do dote on you, but don't be that guy/gal that walks around feeling entitled to it. Remember, there is always someone out there who's worse off than you.

Make sure you ask all these questions before you start treatment because once you start, I can tell you it won't be long before chemo brain sets in, which is this nice, foggy kind of Alzheimer-y thing. You think you're on top of things, but your brain will derail mid-thought. You'll look at people you know well and totally forget their names, or pull up to your house and realize you just did something with the garage door clicker, but no clue what, even though it was just seconds ago you had it in your hand...only to find you didn't actually have it in your hand seconds before because you set it down at the checkout counter at the grocer about an hour before.

You think I'm exaggerating for comedic effect? True story. Another time, I nearly pulled away from the gas pump while the nozzle was still in my tank. Luckily, the guy in the car behind me honked several times. Unluckily, the owner came running out and threatened to charge me a thousand dollars if I had driven off and ruined his pump. I was blonde at the time. This is clue number one why the Ali character on the first book (and the real Ali then) had dark hair.

We all have this spaciness to some degree, but chemo enhances it big time. Blonde or not, you will become a great argument for those jokes. I was visiting a good friend in Ireland last year and her brother (who was unaware of my condition), kept making dumb blonde references. I never corrected him. It would've offended me a decade ago, but honestly, in that moment, I loved it. It was refreshing not to have the dark cloud of cancer over our heads. In that moment, I realized that I'd gladly take dumb blonde over chemo brain as a personal label any day.

I'll talk about it more in the following chapters, but another question between you, yourself, your doc and your boss (if you're currently working) is, "Should I go on medical leave?" A lot of this depends on your treatment plan. The standard medical leave in the US is 90 days. After that, the company is no longer obligated to hold your current position open for you. If your treatment is under 90 days and you love your job, work with them to get coverage while you're out. Chemo treatments are usually set up for every other week, so there is the potential to work on the "off" week, depending on how quickly you can bounce back, or how flexible your boss is about working from home, but listen to me carefully. This is no time to be a workaholic.

That was my MO, and if it wasn't for workmates that were absolute and insistent, I would've tried to stay on, and failed miserably at it. Besides a faltering brain, your body is extremely susceptible to germs and other things that could kill you in your weakened state, so if being in the office is a must, then you have your answer. Bear in mind too, whoever you work for is trying to run a business, and no matter how much they want to accommodate you, they do have a company to run, so don't take their suggestions of backing away or bowing out personally.

If medical leave is the case, then you need to check with your HR department to see what your supplemental disability insurance covers (please for the love of Pete, tell me you have some). State disability is pretty fair, but it's still only about 60 percent of your salary, and it's temporary (in most cases the max is two years). If you're anything like me, that's tough to manage. Learning to adjust to a significant dip in income is a challenge for sure, and believe me, any stress is a bad thing for you right now, so start paring down expenses and ask yourself if continuing to work is going to help you on this road, or hurt you. Only you really know the answer to that.

On to the body...before you start treatment you'll be getting a port implanted. No, I'm not talking about the kind of port that comes in bottles or the one ships sail into, though those are both lovely. This will be the shortest subject because there's not much to say on the matter. You need one. You'll get one. You'll eventually forget you have it, and then one day they'll remove it. It may all seem weird at first, but trust me, before you know it you'll be so glad you have one. I didn't have much time to get used to the idea of having one. I think I underwent the procedure about a week after they told me I needed one, then just a few days after that I started chemo.

A port is this little thing they implant just under the skin in your chest (sometimes arm or abdomen) that has a tube running from it to a major vein. It's where they draw your blood for weekly labs, and it is the entry port for the chemo to get into your system. It may seem icky, but it beats getting poked in the arm or hand every week. Now, there's something to be thankful for. At least you didn't get cancer before they invented the port~

How do I describe a port? It's like one of those rubber balls that glows in the dark and bounces off the walls, but it's cut in half and hollowed out. A tube is attached to one end, and the other end is attached to a major vein. The surgeon creates a little pocket inside the skin for it to sit in; it's all just under the skin. You can barely see mine, where some have a small bump. People always hesitate when I offer to let them touch it, but they say it's kind of cool. Mostly, the scar on the neck shows where they attached it to my jugular, but that's only visible if you're standing pretty close.

I asked Dr. C. (who installed mine), how long I would have it in my body. He shrugged his unworried shoulders, and told me that some patients have kept theirs in for over ten years. I don't know if that's necessary after long term remission, since most places that draw blood won't use it. They have to use a special needle to access it (nah, it doesn't hurt), and they're a lot more expensive than the regular kind. At some point, after you're done with treatment and in the clear, you should have it removed. I wanted to have mine removed before the first book was published, thus reinforcing the validity of the statement, "I beat cancer," as opposed to, "I'm beating cancer." Dr. H. convinced me however, that waiting a year wasn't such a bad idea. If nothing else, it would be nice to give my body a break from anything medically invasive.

I'm so glad I took his advice, and here's mine: Keep it in there because if you fall out of remission and have to go back on chemo, you will have to have a new one implanted, and that will suck. Keep it in at least until you've hit your 5 year anniversary of being in remission. In most cases once you reach that mark, you're supposedly in the clear for good, so what better way to mark the occasion? Pay attention to the "supposedly," though. There are still some docs out there that would say after 5 years, "Good luck, good bye and go have a good life." I currently get scans every 3 months. Once I hit 5 years of remission, then I'll agree to once a year, but I'd never go more than a year without a scan. That's just playing Russian Roulette. Now, I like Russia. I like Vodka even, but I don't like putting a virtual gun to my head and potentially undoing all the hard work it took to get to these extra leases on life

Back to the beginning. I'm not sure if it helps to hear all this beforehand, or if it's better to just go in blind, but I think it would've helped me to understand what was happening well in advance, instead of moments before the procedure. Again, I was on happy pills, so who knows? This is considered an outpatient procedure, so you'll check into the hospital outpatient surgery, and a nice nurse will keep your mind occupied with chitchat, while prepping you for it. The nurse will show you what a port looks like, mentally walk you through how it's implanted, and how it'll work. It looks like a harmless toy. The nurse will also show you the type of needle used to access it during your treatment. The odd thing about the procedure is you'll be awake. Don't worry. You are fully, and I mean fully anesthetized, and you have a big blue sheet above your face, so you don't see any of the gruesomeness, but it was a bit freaky/odd to be talking away with Dr. C. and the nurses, while I couldn't see them.

For some reason, I could feel blood dripping down my neck, but there was no pain, I swear. Even after it all, I didn't feel much of any pain in the incision areas. Some others will disagree, like a guy I know. We'll call him "Gorilla." He implied my statement of, "It didn't hurt," was misleading, and said he was really sore (the weenie), so let's just say, "It could be sore for a week or two while it heals." I kid. He's brave, for a guy ;).

Ok, good to know ahead of time; you have to have someone take you home from the hospital. They won't let you take a cab (I tried), and they're on to all the ways patients try to pretend they have a ride, and then drive themselves home. Pretending your friend is late, and you'll just go wait for them in the cafeteria doesn't fly, trust me. Just face it. This is one of those moments where you gotta let people who love you do their part. Believe it. They want to, so fer fkssake let them help already.

CHAPTER 2
SHOW NO FEAR

🚲 🚲 🚲

This chapter is so important that I bumped it up from Chapter 3, to 2. I've said it before and I'll say it again (and again), cancer is nothing more than a bully. It goes around kicking the crap out of your healthy cells until they give in and join its gang or die trying to defend themselves. I strongly believe it feeds on fear anxiety and repression. You know there's a grain of truth to all those sayings like, "She was worried sick," and "That guy needs to calm down. He's a heart attack waiting to happen."

So, how do you beat a bully? You can pretend to ignore it or at least refuse to give it credence for starters. I used to do this by refusing to capitalize its name. That may seem silly, but the mind is a very powerful thing, and every time I used a lowercase letter, I imagined it shrinking in strength. I've gotten over that now, and just don't give it much of my attention, ccapitalized or not. Sometimes, I still flip it the bird when I hear it mentioned on TV or radio, but usually to myself, or under the table when in public. No big scene.

For decades now, we've cowered at the mention of it, and understandably so, but modern medicine is catching up to cancer, so should our perception of it. Back in the early 90's when my mother had cancer, no one had even heard of targeted radiation therapy or radio surgery, but in 2011 that is exactly what they did to fix my left lung. Today, there are several different brands of it, but all result in the same thing; non invasive targeted killing of cancer cells. Just three years later, I went through another type of targeted radiation therapy on a spot that formed in my right lung. In 2011, they injected gold flecks in my lung as markers. With this one, they used tiny tattooed dots as markers. This is how I discovered that tattoos are indeed painful...I have thus scratched, "get a tattoo," off my bucket list. I call my little group of dots my "constellation" tattoo, or "connect the dots" tattoo, whenever someone asks if I have one.

Seriously though, without those therapies I wouldn't be alive today because chemo shrunk them, but never completely rid my body of them. Again, I'm not trying to give anyone false hope. I just think it's time we recognize the vast improvements that have happened, move beyond the darker images and gut-wrenching emotions from the days of *Terms of Endearment* and face these little feckers, armed with determination, and the latest greatest information available. Maybe then, we can finally relegate it to the ranks of other diseases that are mere shadows in history.

So, the first step in fighting back is showing no fear. When people around you are afraid for you, reassure them you're not afraid and they shouldn't be either. I know, I know. You ARE afraid. Trust me when I tell you that you must stop that right now.

Do whatever it takes to find your happy place and/or fake it till you make it, baby. Your life may very well depend on it. It's the simple equation of this; If stress and depression are damaging and positive energy is healing, then doesn't it make sense that the more positive energy you emit the greater the chances of survival?

Hey, If that's too Pollyanna for you, then I'll go darker. What if you don't make it? What if you've got a year left in this life? Do you really want to spend it buried under a pile of stress and regrets or would you rather spend it laughing, loving and enjoying life? I'll give you two guesses what my choice was and still is after years of this cancer crap...

I have done more traveling and taken more risks since I was diagnosed than I have in my entire life. I've found that reaching out and getting more of what I really want out of life is so much easier than holding back and regretting missed opportunities. I still have a ways to go in some areas. It is harder to let new people into your life when you worry about how the shadow of your illness will affect your relationship, but it's important to remember that it is their choice to make. A hard one for me too, but a must. What's the point of working so hard to stay alive if you're not going to fully live? And to fully live you must engage with other people. Not all people, mind you. Some are just soul suckers, so don't waste your time on those, but you know what I'm saying.

This brings to mind a moment with my sister. For some reason, I was determined to jump in a lake on my birthday this year. Every birthday now, I feel a strong urge to either do something that scares me or something I've always wanted to do. Jumping in a lake features both. What's so scary about a lake? Fear of drowning and creatures of the black lagoon come to mind. For some reason, sometimes I forget to breathe right, and I'm afraid I'll forget to hold my breath when I dive in. I never fail to do so, but I seem to have developed a fear I will, this one time, and how ironic that would be if that's how I eventually died. "It wasn't the cancer that killed her. The idiot forgot to hold her breath when she jumped in the water..."

Anyway, we were at a beautiful place called Lake Arrowhead. Standing on the dock, I slowly stripped down to my swimsuit and tried to distract her with nonsensical chatter, then I stood at the end and just stared into the darkness below...I saw my reflection, some green slime on the ladder that I'd be climbing up out of the water from, and some bits of stuff floating around. I wondered if my white blood cell count was high enough to ward off any buggers that might infiltrate my body once submerged. I'd forgotten how murky lakes can be... I stood there for the longest time, when she asked if I was going to jump in or not. I stepped back. I knew she could see how nervous I was, but she didn't look annoyed so much as confused. I mean, I talked about it for months like a little kid counting down the days till Christmas...

Finally, she said, "If I jump in with you will you do it?" I reluctantly agreed, and on the count of 3 we jumped in (though I lagged a second behind her to make sure she actually did it). It was actually, really refreshing. She even suggested we make it an annual thing, which I love. To anyone else, this might all seem like such a mountain made from a mole hill, but never forget that what may seem insignificant to you may be monumental to another, and it's quite possibly a pivotal moment for them, if they could push through it. One less thing to be afraid of, that's the way to see it.

It's funny how in that moment we take things to heart, but the very next day we can just as easily fall back into our somewhat deluded perception that life goes on and it's business as usual. Even with all I've experienced these past few years, I still have moments where I get caught up in the dramas of day-to-day life, and little annoyances drive my temper to a boil, or I shrink back with trepidation. Human nature is such a wild and beguiling mystery at times. Will that particular piece of the puzzle be solved once we reach the other side? I am curious...but am in absolutely no rush to find out.

So, we touched on it, but we have to go there if we're really going to show NO fear. If this is news to you, then I'm sorry to be the one to break it to you, but you ARE going to die. Well, you are going to die one day, that is. Unless you are immortal, and it's yet to be proven that anyone is, then we all are going to croak/kick the bucket at some point. If you haven't accepted it yet, then get over it already and stop watching stupid movies like *Final Destination XXI,* that portray death as some vindictive b@stard that will chase you down and make you pay in the worst way if you dare attempt to cheat it. Death isn't sporting for a brawl, or some psycho killer on the loose, randomly striking people down for sport.

Also, fer fkssake, you did NOT get cancer because you bullied that other kid in grade school and never made amends. Neither cancer, nor death, is punishment, but a means to an end. It is cause and effect, if you will. You are born, so therefore at some point you'll die. At least your body does. My take on it? I think that as long as there is something or someone to remember you by, then you never completely cease to exist. My stories, books and music are my way of sticking around long after my body goes kaput. I get that from my mom. She made sure each of us had a quilt especially made for us by her. Each unique in its own way, and definitely makes me think of her every time I see it.

As for the, "Why me?" Does it really matter how you got cancer right now? You can dig and research from here to Timbuktu and back, but it's not going to change the fact you have cancer. I stand by the point to leave it, for now, to the experts to discover causes and cures, and spend your energy on situations you can take charge of. It's there, and it's not going away on its own, so think of this as a gentle reminder that you are going to die, at some point. If your life got off track from what you wanted it to be, take this momentous opportunity to get it back on track. Once all the dust has settled and your head stops spinning, then yes, it's always good to be actively involved in your treatment.

With every passing year, there are more and more options out there for treating each specific cancer. It's good to be aware of your options and to partner with your providers in deciding how best to attack it.

Even if you're not prone to anxiety or depression, you may want to consider going on something during the duration of your treatment. I highly recommend it (no pun intended). I went with Welbutron (Bupropion) for the first year because from what I'd read, it seemed the simplest. It was like the aspirin of antidepressants. I'm not keen on the fancier new meds, with all their bells and whistles. I had to skip the night dosage (it kept me wiiiide awake), but other than that, I felt no side effects. It was just a nice little wave of calm that washed over me whenever the anxiety tried to well up.

Don't dig taking a pill? Then, check with a naturopath or the cool lady at the health-food store for a natural supplement. Every body and mind is different, so find whatever works best for you, but be sure to consult with your cancer doc, before spending any money on remedies.

After the first year of treatment, I weaned myself off the antidepressants and experimented with natural solutions like; B complex, L-Glutamine and Primrose Oil with Black Cohosh. I don't know which one works better, since I take them all daily, and have for quite a while now, but they all have made a difference in several ways, and it goes along nicely with my *nuture with nature* frame of mind.

Whatever you do, don't be naive in thinking you've got all the raw positive energy needed to deal with this. Pollyanna may be my middle name, and though I took my happy pills religiously, I still had my dark moments. Why suffer unnecessarily? This is all tough enough as it is.

So, let's say it: "SHOW NO FEAR" Go ahead, say it like

you mean it, and then, mean it. I even use this saying when I'm facing day to day fears, like just as I'm stepping up to a microphone, or the time when my tour guide pushed my sea kayak out into the waters of La Jolla Cove and toward the scary waves (whopping two-footers). I said it under my breath so as not to appear too dorky, but I said it with true conviction. It feels really good I'm telling you~

So, here's where I hope you are now. You know what your treatment plan is, and you have an added boost (herbal or RX) to help you keep in calm waters through it all. You are FEARLESS, and ready to take on the next addition to your arsenal. Time to check out those silver linings...

CHAPTER 3
THE UPSIDE (OR EVERY CLOUD HAS ITS SILVER LINING)

🚲 🚲 🚲

In the first book I shared a story about my friend Jen, who is a shining example of someone who weathers the storms, and is one of the first to see the ray of light ahead.

In the last few years, she has lost her mom to cancer, lost her nephew to sudden death, and gained a new last name, but almost lost her newlywed husband to a massive stroke. She also pushed herself through an intensive training course to become a nurse, thus the new nick, "Jen RN." There were a few times that Jen nearly lost herself in the madness, but somehow she pulled through.

Jen and I have a similar outlook on life. We tend to take on others' burdens, but we also have an enormous capacity for love. When we take on too much crap, it bogs us down, we get overwhelmed and well, bitchy (I can spell this one out because it's not technically a swear). Jen RN has had every reason to be bitchy, but some kind of switch flips in her before it gets too dark. She sees and focuses on the silver lining. You have those friends, right? They are great at helping you put things back into perspective, and allowing you to do the same for them, when they need it.

I called her up to go over the changes to this chapter, and making sure I got it all right. She gently explained to me the difference between an aneurism (which I originally wrote had happened to her husband), and a stroke (what actually happened to her husband). Then we went on to talk about my recent health updates, and the differences between the various cancer centers in our area. She explained that one nearest her, baked cookies on a daily basis. I said, "Doesn't that go against all the hype about sugar being bad for you if you have cancer?" She responded (as only Jen RN can), "Are you kidding me? You've got fkn cancer. Have a cookie!"

Jen and I run the gambit whenever we talk, just as our brains do. You know how I say that nobody really ceases to exist, as long as there is something or someone around to remember them by? I'm not sure how we got onto this topic, but Jen has settled in the field of Oncology. The same field her mom was in, for the last decade of her career/life. Jen says, she feels it's where her heart is. How many can say that about the job they are doing?

Anyway, Jen was talking about how she'd been holding onto her mom's nursing scrubs. That she and her mom were a different build, so even though Jen had lost a lot of weight over the past year, and was at a good and healthy weight, her mom's scrubs still didn't fit her, so she brought them into work at the hospital, put them in the staff lounge with a note; welcoming anyone to take them and put them to good use. "Every now and then, I'll see a nurse walk by me and I think; Hey, those are mom's scrubs. Hi mom." I could feel her smile coming through the phone line, and I just love how I could envision exactly what she was describing.

Every time I talk to Jen, I'm reminded of how unpredictable life is, and how lucky I am to have so many good people to go through it with.

We all have our freak-out moments, and we're allowed them, but don't forget to shift to the lighter side of it when you're done. Yes, you have it bad. You may even have the worst case of cancer, since the inception of cancer. Maybe, they're thinking of renaming your type of cancer after you because it's so rare, mystifying and devastating. Okay, okay.

Just remember; no matter how bad you've got it, someone else out there has it worse.

There are people, other than yourself, who are piecing their lives back together after surviving; a devastating tsunami, earthquake or mudslide. There are so many wounded warriors among us, learning to live on with physical limitations, and struggling to quiet their minds from PTSD. And how about Bethany Hamilton? At the tender age of 13, she was out surfing when she was attacked by a shark, losing her left arm. This girl could've given up, but instead, she got back on her surfboard just a month later. Two years after that, she won first place in the NSSA National Championships.

These people are clear examples of how to persevere and get on with life. To quote one of my favorite Japanese proverbs, "Fall down 7 times, stand up 8." That type of mentality is what you need to grab hold of and mind meld with (that one's for you, dear Spock). Of course, it's ok to feel down sometimes from all of this. Just don't let it suck you into that long dark tunnel, cutting you off from the rest of the world, or the amazing-ness it offers up on a silver platter, nearly every day. Take a moment, then get back up, dust yourself off, and get back to living.

Speaking of silver linings, here's an update to the original story of Jen RN, in the first book. Since *The C Card and Me* was published in 2012, there's a new niece in Jen's life, and a nephew on the way. She says, her family are all turning their heads toward her and her husband (who is nearly 100% recovered, thank you very much). To which, she'd like to say, "Take a pic it'll last longer." They are enjoying and allowing themselves to soak in this time of even keel in their lives. Good for them.

I love to "fix" broken things, and improve situations in need.

I thrive on it. When people ask me, "What makes you happy?" I say, "Being useful." Every time I get positive feedback from readers, or hear that someone is passing on something they found helpful from the book, I feel useful. I feel like I'm earning my keep in this world.

Being diagnosed with cancer (regardless of what stage), dramatically changes your perspective on life. This is a golden opportunity to find and take stock in your own personal silver linings. Do you remember the road trip game we'd play as kids? You'd call out, "red car," and then we'd all call out a red car when we saw one. Suddenly, it seemed like there were so many red cars on the road. Well, it's like that, only I'm calling out, "Silver linings~"

On to the funnest topic ever, money matters…

CHAPTER 4
SHOW ME THE MONEY

🚲 🚲 🚲

This was probably the toughest one for me. Some have it tougher; some need not give it a thought. This chapter is dedicated to those whose hearts start to race every time they pull a bill out of the postbox, and are slightly freaked at the thought of managing to pay for all this life-saving treatment, and still keep a roof over their heads.

I know that donations have helped medical science make great strides in the search for a cure and in treatment, but the those big-name cancer charities that you walk for days for, or dress to show unity with, don't help individual patients grapple with the crushing debt, that is the exchange for life saving treatment. And it's moments like these, when you are staring at a $16,000 medical bill, you begin to ask yourself, if those alternative sources might be the better way to go. Whatever you do, do NOT let the high cost be the reason you don't do chemo.

Oh, if I could rule the world. I would declare that all life saving treatments must be made affordable, based on the patient's ability to pay. I would ensure that there were medical billing expert/advocates on hand, who could help each patient decipher all the garble that goes into their bills, and that everything is billed correctly. Y'see, on top of the stress and general suckiness of chemo, you have to comb through your medical bills because surprisingly, more often than expected, they will be incorrect. At least, that is my case and the case of the patients I've spoken to. I've switched insurance plans three times since I started treatment in 2010. The first plan was through my employer, the second was on Medicare, with an IPA that treated people like cattle, and the third is still Medicare with an IPA that is on top of everything, but billing. So, nearly a year after treatment, I received a bill for over $16,000, with very few details, other than it was apparently for one cycle of chemo (remember, I've had over 40 cycles and about 8 with this current plan). When I called, they said it was indeed incorrect, and was more like $1,000 per cycle. Funny, because with the previous insurance plan, I was paying about $200 per cycle. Now, I'll tell you this before I rant on any further. I used to work in the medical field. I had friends who worked in the billing department, and they would often lament how difficult it is to keep up with all of the codes. I get that it isn't an easy task, so let's not go postal on the billing people.

Just do yourself a favor. When you get that bill, take a deep breath and tell yourself, "You are not bigger than me." Say that whenever anything overwhelms you. It's okay to shed a few tears of frustration. You never want to bottle that stuff up or it'll fester, but let them roll down your face and say those words to whatever is troubling you, "You are not bigger than me." It really works. After years of this, and what some would consider crippling debt, my head is still above water because I just keep plugging away at it.

Writing this reminds me of a good friend of mine who used to run a local pub/restaurant. At the time I'm thinking of, the city had suddenly spiked the rates for electricity. The local businesses were balking at it, and some even refused to pay their bills entirely (out of protest). She chose to call them, and calmly discuss a payment plan. People were surprised that she didn't rebel and kick up a fuss, but she knew…"This too shall pass." When other businesses had to close because their power had been turned off, her lights were on. She was still in business. The point of the story? Keep your lights on. No one says you have to pay this huge pile off all at once, or even in big chunks. They care more that you are consistent in payments than how much is coming in. Paying $100/month on $18,000 (or more) in medical debt, will not mean two guys in ski masks will be pounding down your door with a baseball bat. These are not loan sharks. These are cancer centers, and most are well funded. They will send you to collections if you don't pay anything, and that means your credit score will plummet. You don't want that.

Keeping your score up means a financial cushion that you could use later for rent/mortgage, or maybe even checking something off your bucket list. Believe me, the well will, at some point, run dry on financial support, so you need to be smarter than ever about money.

When it comes to your credit, bear in mind these two things; nearly 1/3 of your credit score is based on how much of the available credit you use, and late payments count for almost another 1/3 of your score. Remember these two things to keep your credit rating decent during this time. Try your best to not to use more than half your available credit (If you have $2,000 in credit, never use up more than $1,000). That isn't on each card. It means your total, so you could rack up 70% on one and 30% on another and still be only using 50% of your "overall" credit. To keep from being late, setup automatic payments on all your debts, to pay at least the minimum. The minimum plus is better (even if it's just by a few bucks). Late payments will stay on your credit report for 7 years. That's a long time for a totally avoidable pain in the arse.

I was lucky to find a volunteer advocate who helped me enormously. She told me about several local resources for financial support, went through my day-to-day expenses, and showed me where I could cut back (at least temporarily). In the end, she saved me a lot of money and more importantly, stress.

There was still a pile of bills, but at least it was a manageable one. Through cancer support resources, you can find; reimbursement for gas, groceries, co-payments, and insurance premiums. There are even some places that offer transportation to/from chemo and house cleaning services. Even with all the help though, you still have to pay attention. Having chemo brain (we've discussed), meant I made more mistakes on forms and account updates than I care to admit. When that happens, be sure to whip out your c card. Some people forget there's another human being on the other end of the line. A gentle reminder of your condition can change that tone and often the outcome of the conversation.

All said and done, my out-of-pocket expenses have come out to about 10K per year of treatment, so far, which is a lot to some and not much to others. For me, it meant putting some dreams on hold and scaling down others. I could fill a hundred pages with all the great things my friends and family did for me through all of this (despite my resistance), but the important message you need to hear is that when your friends and family volunteer to help, you say, "THANK YOU." Know that by letting them help you, are helping them deal. Face it, oh defiant one, you need the help.

You know, they say don't expect it, but I'll bet if you allow it to happen, when it comes your way, you'll be surprised and touched by the generosity of others, and sometimes it's from those you'd least expect. Okay, that's enough mush. Let's get back to your insider's guide.

First, a note to those who don't have to give a thought to the money side. Have a think on this...as you go through this course of treatment (or you are holding the hand of someone who is), you are going to witness loads of people who don't have it quite so good. No doubt, your money is your own and you've earned every bit of it. Why should you give any of it to someone who didn't plan ahead, or work as smart as you? You should because even if you have the equivalent value of the crown jewels in your bank account, this ride can be a burden on the soul. The joy you can get from seeing relief on a stranger's face can easily increase those mighty mind and body-healing endorphins, and there is no better time to stock up on those good karma points~

Next, let's get it all out in the open...

CHAPTER 5
LAY YOUR CARDS ON THE TABLE

🚲 🚲 🚲

I was pretty protective of my privacy during the first year or so, but there was one thing I did in the very beginning, when rumors were flying, and people didn't know what (if anything) to say. I don't know if this was the best way to do it, but it was my way.

I started off by sending a group e-mail to most of my local friends. These were the ones who'd see me face-to-face, while this was all happening. It was an up-front, no-holds-barred e-mail. It was the first time I wrote out the words "Stage IV," and it shook me up a bit, but I knew I had to tell them all the same story. It had to be the true story, all at once, if I was to get any peace. They were, after all, already assuming the worst. Plus, I wanted to be sure it stayed off my personal, social media. I wanted to keep that place lighthearted with all the bantering and social escapes it offered. "Hey everybody. I've got cancer and it's Stage IV~" just didn't seem the kind of status update Facebook was designed for.

In the email, I told them my prognosis, the plan, and what I needed from them. First and foremost, I needed them not to worry. I went on to explain that when they worried, I stressed out because I didn't want them to worry, which meant their worrying and stress impeded my healing process, so it would actually be detrimental to me if they worried.

I also asked them not to treat me like I was sick. "If you treat me like I'm dying I'll feel like I'm dying," I said. I told them I would be going on with life and enjoying many of the same things, and some new ones, just in smaller doses, reserving most of my energy for the treatments and recovery.

I laughed and flirted with my docs, and befriended my nurses (which was really easy, by the way). They were all so very cool. Smiling, laughing, flirting, and joking...these all increase the endorphins in your body, and we all know endorphins are a good thing. I envisioned the endorphins as little rays of sunbeams, blasting light onto the dark matter (another word I use for cancer cells) lurking around in my body.

The last thing I said, was that I wanted them to feel free to talk about it openly, to me or amongst themselves. I wasn't trying to keep this a deep, dark secret. I wanted it to become matter-of-fact. When you tell people you've got cancer, they tend to want to give you the shirt off their back, even when it isn't necessary. It made me uncomfortable, and I know this may sound strange, but I sort of felt like they'd be disappointed if I got well, after all the fuss they'd gone to. Then again, maybe it was just me on that one.

Oh, I couldn't resist. I did make a point to my smoking friends. I wasn't going to judge or harp on them, but they should probably pay close attention to the details of the treatments (crap) I was going through. They'd probably be needing that info for future reference. What, I already admitted I can be kind of a brat sometimes.

Looking back, I do regret this part, so heed my warning. There were some people back home...I never told. I didn't exclude anyone out of malice or lack of regard. Oddly enough, the ones I didn't tell were because I thought they would worry the most, and I couldn't stand the thought of it. I even lied to my dad, and said it was just a tumor. This is a baaad idea peeps. Eventually, someone (like, I don't know, say, maybe your sister) is going to slip up/spill the beans, and it'll make those people you didn't the whole story to, worry all the more. After all, if you lied about that, what else are you not telling them?

It's a lot of pressure to put on someone, to keep a secret like that. It's also kind of unfair, don't you think? Do you see how best intentions are good to scrutinize after putting them in motion? I need a full-time person for that, let me tell you.

Okay, so all your loved ones are in the know, and clear on what you need. What's next? Time to get your clean on...

CHAPTER 6
THINK SPRING CUZ IT'S TIME TO CLEAN

🚲 🚲 🚲

Even if your prognosis is rosy, if you haven't already, you might as well buck up and get that last W&T put together. You may not have a pot to piss in, but believe it or not, there are things of yours that loved ones will consider of great value to them, and they'll want to hold onto them, to remember you by.

Save those you leave behind the hassle, and put together a will. Update it every now and then, when your list of valuables changes. This also helps keep you grounded in the reality that you are not immortal, and you should live every day to the fullest.

Another element to the whole embracing life thing, is to stop doing the stupid things that just beg for serious health troubles. We all have our vices and we all know which ones are really hurting us, so you'll get no pointing of fingers or lecturing here. I'll just out myself on this one, alright?

Now, anyone who knows me, considers me a *Pollyanna,* of sorts (I have my dark moments too), but what many (and I'm still surprised by this) didn't know, is that I have always been anxious. It was big smiles on the outside but shaking like a Chihuahua on the inside. My mind would hyper-analyze whatever I was about to deal with, till my heart felt it would nearly burst out of my chest, and then I'd light up a cig and breathe in…breathe out…and calm myself. That's how I dealt with it for nearly twenty years. I'd light up a cig every time I felt it creeping on, which added up to anywhere between a pack, to two packs a day. Okay, yes, I also used them to manage my weight because if you didn't catch it before, I love to eat. Look up "ultimate foodie" in the dictionary, and my picture should be there with Bolognese sauce around the corners of my mouth.

When it was clear I was in some kind of serious health trouble, I asked my doc for a prescription to help curb my anxiety (the trigger), so I could kick the twenty-something-year habit. After all, it seemed ludicrous (even to my thick head) to expect the doctors to fix me, when I was doing plenty of damage on my own. Like a bad, but horribly attractive ex, I miss cigarettes to this day, yet I got it, there had to be some compromise on my part.

More than that though, I had to take part in the healing. I couldn't leave all the work up to the doctors and nurses, if I really expected to take any credit for my recovery, and so, that was it. That was in April of 2010, and by that September, I had undergone the surgery to remove the tumor in my colon (charmingly referred to as a Sigmoidectomy). I have no doubt that I recovered from it much faster than if I'd still been a smoker.

Okay, I can be a bit of a jerk when it comes to friends who still smoke. I won't stand by them when they do, which breaks up the momentum of our conversations, and that annoys them, I can tell. Guess what? It totally fekkn annoys me that you don't get how much shite I've gone through, and how much shite you're going to go through because you are standing in the same line I was, and that means you are headed toward the same fate. The only winners in this are the tobacco companies, who love the fact that they've lulled us into forgetting we're paying good money to breath in something that damages us.

It's easy to forget how harmful they are. I recently met up with a friend I hadn't seen in years. As we were walking the streets of Manhattan, he asked (polite as always) if I minded if he lit up. I said in my most adorable tone "No, no, not at all," when what I wanted to say was, "Are you feckn kidding me?" Or, maybe I should've used the line that an old beau once said to me, "Hey, it's your lungs you're killing, not mine."

I was really enjoying what felt like a normal, cancer free moment and he is so damned handsome...I lost myself for a moment, so if you are reading this, and you know me, or ever run into me, know this...YES, I mind if you smoke. Not because I'm an ex-smoking snob, but because I genuinely do not want you to have to go through all the crappy things one has to go through to beat cancer. Wake up, and smell the nicotine that's infiltrating your system. I know, it made me feel cool too, and definitely made keeping my weight in-check easier, but the payback's a bitch and a half. You, continuing to smoke after reading this, is like standing on one end of a fire pouring kerosene about while firefighters on the other end are trying to put it out.

But, let's end this chapter on a more positive note. Get out the ole calculator and figure out how much you spend on cigs each day, then times it by 352 (because riiiight...you don't smoke every day of the year). Now, start listing all the amazingly cool things you could do with that money. Mine was enough for a trip abroad, per year. Now, how many times in the last couple decades (when I was earning nearly six figures) did I say I wanted to go to Europe, but didn't have the money? Chew on that.

Right, then. Time to get a bigger boat...

CHAPTER 7
WE'RE GOING TO NEED A BIGGER BOAT (EH MEDICINE CABINET)

🚲 🚲 🚲

That's right. If you haven't already, head into your bathroom with a garbage bag, and throw out all the crap in the medicine cabinet (diet pills, outdated prescriptions and anything else you don't use). I'd be surprised if you'll even be able to close the cabinet door, once you're done filling it with your new arsenal of feel-good items. I made a friend at chemo in the first year, after I'd gotten into the swing of things. It was her first day, and I surprised myself, how I couldn't stop talking about all the things I wish I'd known on my first day. I promised to make her a list of medicine cabinet items she'd need. I think that's when the seed was planted to write the first cancer survival guide.

Side effects...this is a tough one to cover because there are so many, and they vary, depending on what type of cancer you have. Believe it or not, there are many different types of cancer (over 100), and different types of drug treatments which have different side effects. A common misconception (that I had up until the day of my orientation), was that all cancer patients lose their hair. This is no longer true. It is still a side-effect of the drugs used to treat cancers in reproductive areas (and possibly others, but I'm no expert on that). If they tell you, you're going to lose your hair, you're either going to shrug because you don't mind (or you're already bald), or if it were me, I'd shrug my shoulders and say, "cool." That would mean you'd get to try a bunch of different hair colors and styles you wouldn't normally go for. Silver linings...

Going bald was not a side effect I experienced. Instead (probably because I was already hypothyroid), I gained well (and I mean weeeeell) over fifty pounds in the year and a half of treatment. I complained at every sitting with Dr. H., but he just gave me a blank stare. Sometimes, a sigh of exhaustion slid under it as he reminded me; weight gain is not a matter of concern. Each time, he'd say this with increasing emphasis until he finally pointed out the sad fact that he had some patients, who were so thin, he could actually see their organs bulging through their concave bellies (i.e., Ali...we've got bigger fish to fry than your vanity's struggle over weight gain).

I tried my best to avoid that subject from then on, but the broken record continued to play on in my head. Every time I'd mention it to my friend Jen, who was studying to be a nurse at the time, she'd remind me it was a good thing. It would help my body fight the good fight. I don't even care if that's true. I loved her for saying it because it DID make me feel better about it. It's ironic, don't you think? There I was, skating along the edge of life or death and I couldn't stop lamenting over weight gain. Ohhh, the mighty mind versus the whimpering ego.

Another side effect you can't treat with meds, is sensitivity to light and sun. This is where you'll break out in bumps and sometimes blisters, from what you'd consider normal exposure to the sun. If this is one of your side effects just wear sun protective clothing, and at least SPF 50 on any exposed skin. It's important to get your natural doses of vitamin D, just keep that sun exposure to snippets of time. I can tell you, I did NOT listen to that advice very well, and during one of my breaks I thought I would be fine in the sun. It had been at least a couple weeks since my last chemo session, so no problem, right? We had another one of our friends' day outings. About sixteen of us hopped on our beach cruisers and did a house crawl. We stopped at each of our houses (there were seven within a three-mile radius), and at each one, was a different food/drink served. I made homemade blueberry and cranberry muffins, and mimosas with grapefruit, cranberry and lemon (ever the hostess with the mostess).

What, I was on a break. So, it went on from noon till sundown, when we met up at the last house, grilled, and sat around a bonfire. See…this is what I mean by enjoying life. Though my lovely and protective friends all took turns spraying me head-to-toe throughout the day, we did miss a spot…the lips. Even with my baseball cap on all day, they managed to get burnt. They were crispy, blistery, thoroughly painful, and embarrassingly icky looking, which lasted well over a week. So please, for the love of Pete, take heed. These are pearls I'm giving you. Pearls, I tell ye~

Another side effect is sensitivity to cold. This one, I shrugged off, when they told me. Even as I started chemo, I thought it was minor, at worst. I was not thinking it was cumulative, as in; the more chemo you get, the stronger the side effect becomes and the longer it lingers. A couple of months into it, I had to wear gloves at night, if there was any hint of chill in the air. The cool air bit like it was winter in the frozen tundra. That wasn't the worst of it though. Any surface, such as; a car door handle, fridge, or microwave, felt like touching dry ice. The trick, was to wear long-sleeve shirts, and pull the bottom of the sleeve over your hand before touching anything like that. I don't care if it's August, and blazing heat is running through your home, don't even think about trying to eat or drink anything straight from the fridge, or even something that's so-called, "room temperature." It's like swallowing an ice cube.

One other side effect worth mentioning, is that cotton mouth/chemical thing that lines the inside of your mouth and sinuses. I'm pretty sure everyone gets to experience this lovely one. You can rinse to get rid of the cotton, but the chemical ick taste will stick and anything milder than Vindaloo or five alarm chili will taste just plain ole weird. I've said it a couple times in this book, but I'll say it again; avoid all the foods and beverages you love. If you don't, they will forever be ruined by the chemical ick. Stick to spicy and citrus flavors. Sometimes, eating sliced cucumber, or drinking sparkling mineral water (with lemon) helped too .

Let's go back to the cabinet. I made a list. Now, these are the side effects I dealt with. There are other ones out there, but these, I can tell you about, first hand. Keep this list handy. You'll be glad to have it there, at the ready, when your symptoms kick in. Before you go out and buy any of these remedies, be sure to go over the list with your doc and make sure they agree. They're the boss of you. I'm just a friend who's been there.

SIDE EFFECTS AND RELIEVERS

Nausea/Anxiety—Ativan (and Mary Jane).

The runs—Imodium A-D.

To soothe the burning ring of fire—Tucks medicated wipes or Preparation H.

The log jam—Probiotics with at least 50 billion strains will help replenish what's being stripped by chemo. Also MiraLAX (best taken in small doses every day, see recipe below).

Can't sleep—Tylenol PM or Benadryl. Beware; prolonged use of Naproxen can cause stomach ulcers.

Can't stop sniffling—Claritin or NyQuil to sleep through it.

Flu-like symptoms, especially after getting Immune booster shots—Claritin or Benedryl. Take the night before and for four days following the shot.

Bloody nose and dry sinuses—saline spray every morning and night.

Dry mouth/Bleeding gums—softer toothbrush and gentle paste, but they will still bleed until you're no longer anemic. Biotene helps keep balance, but my friend Marlene, who is a dental hygienist recently told me that CloSYS has a, "better PH balance," and that's what you'll need help regaining during chemo She has gorgeous teeth, so I'll give it a try~

Acid reflux—Zantac or the generic version.

Urinary tract infection (UTI) —Drink the cranberry cocktail (see below) at least once a day to keep UTIs at bay, and to HYDRATE.

Sensitivity to sunlight—Always wear at least 50spf sun protection when outside keep exposure to sunlight minimal until at least four weeks after treatment to avoid blistering and rashes.

Gas—Gas-X. You're going to be drawn to spicy foods so trust me. I tried the generic brand. It's not even close to as effective so go for the original. You could also try Beano before you eat.

Mouth sores/thrush—Use equal parts: xylocaine viscous solution, Zovirax (alcohol-free), and Maalox, or Mylanta. Take 2 teaspoons every 2-4 hours as needed (swish around mouth and spit out). Avoid anything with alcohol in it. Also see Mary's advice in chapter 10.

Joint aches —Antler Velvet. I was hard hit by joint aches for months before a friend suggested antler velvet. I tried a couple different brands after, but the purer the better I say. It worked within a couple of short weeks. The pain before was so bad that I kissed the empty bottle before tossing it out.

Joint swelling/edema—flush that system with water and movement. Reduce salt intake and use natural diuretics like tea. Midol (or similar brand) helps too.

Hot flashes—GNC's Phyto-Estrogen Formula (Black Cohosh and Primrose Oil).

You'll also want a thermometer on hand, if you don't already. Having a temperature is a sign of infection, and infections are a very bad thing. You can have one and not even know it, so be sure to take your temp daily when you're not being seen by the pros. Ask them. They'll tell you how often to check.

Anti-UTI/Log Jam Cranberry Cocktail

32-oz bottle of water (suck out ½ cup of it)
¼ cup or more of just cranberry (unsweetened) juice
or add fresh-squeezed lemon or lime to it.
½ cap of MiraLAX and shake it up good.

Mix all ingredient in the bottle. Drink one of these in the morning and one in the afternoon/evening as needed.

Immune Booster Shake

1 cup almond milk
Splash of just cranberry (unsweetened) juice
Dash of ground allspice
Frozen fruit (organic)
1 tsp(ish) of matcha (green tea) powder
Large scoop of plant protein powder
1 tblsp of L-Glutamine powder
Large scoop of plain yogurt
1 raw egg
Splash of sparkling mineral water

Blend it all together and drink every morning before tea or coffee. This combo of antioxidants and probiotics will help boost your immune systems, detox the chemical and rebalance your digestive tract.

Since I started drinking the cranberry cocktail during cycles, I haven't had one UTI, not one. I started drinking those shakes just after the last chemo cycle finished and my chemo break began, when my WBC was 2.9 (4.0-10.0 is normal range). Within a month, my WBC shot up to 4.2, and the next month it was 5.3. It hasn't been that high in years. How's that for pudding proof? Check with your doc, but I'm pretty sure, unless you have sensitivity to cold, you should be able to drink those shakes during a chemo cycle as well. If not, at least during your off week to help boost your levels back up.

I asked the nurses if they had any additional suggestions. Anita mentioned taking thin slices of gingerroot, and either sucking on them or putting them in water, and drinking that to ease nausea. It makes sense. I'm not a fan of fresh ginger though. It tastes like soap to me. The thought of it actually makes me a little nauseous, so I'll be skipping out on that one, but it is a great suggestion. I'm thinking back to how my mom gave us saltine crackers and ginger ale to soothe our tummies, and I remember liking ginger ale, especially the one she grew up with (Vernors), back in Michigan. It's funny how that all ties in together...comfort foods of our youth and the medicinal properties they actually held.

Did I already say; stay away from the foods/beverages you love? Yes, I did. I was just checking to see if you were paying attention. On that note though, there are two kinds of food you need to avoid regardless of your taste buds. These are grapefruit and raw meats/seafood. Avoid grapefruit because it can interfere with the effectiveness of most cancer drugs. Avoid raw meat or seafood (of any kind) because of the bacteria it contains. Your body normally can easily deal with that bacteria, but it's too busy fighting off the other stuff during chemo, so you could get incredibly sick. This is no joke. Stay clear from both. I am a sushi lover. Two years living in Tokyo made me a fan for life, and I was used to eating sushi at least once or twice a week, so say "no" to it was never easy.

I'm also what you might call a grapefruit enthusiast (okay, addict). I could eat/drink the stuff daily. When I was a smoker, I drank a large glass of grapefruit juice almost every day. Someone once pointed out that my body was craving vitamin C because nicotine depletes your body of it. Ohhhh, you will discover many correlations like this. That said, putting aside your favorite foods and beverages can be hard, but man oh man, it tastes so good when you finally get back to them~

Right, then. It's time to meet up with Mary Jane and the gang...

CHAPTER 8
SAY "HEY" TO MARY JANE AND THE GANG

🚲 🚲 🚲

There's been some controversy over this subject, but for the most part (at least in California), we've all gotten over it, and realized though some knuckleheads overuse it to escape reality, it does have its purposes. I'm one of those that believe in *live and let live*, but if it's illegal, I'm going to stay clear of it. You can take the girl out of the Catholic church...

Well, here's another silver lining in your c world. It's now legal for you and most docs even encourage you to make friends with Mary Jane, aka 420, or marijuana, to help keep nausea at bay, and thus maintain a healthy weight. My doctor didn't feel the need to recommend this to me, thanks to my family's policy: eat when you're happy, eat when you're sad, eat when you're sick, and eat even when you're mad. You can get the RX from your oncology or general doc, then you go to this store that offers a plethora of choices. You can smoke it in a pipe, roll it like a cig, or enjoy it in a Rice Krispy treat (go with the edible kind if your lungs are in treatment). You name it. It's all at your disposal, and you should feel free to indulge. A lot of people also use it to treat their anxiety, and swear it works wonders.

Okay, I know you want to ask, "Won't getting this RX put me on some kind of government watch list, or put me at risk for being declined for certain future jobs?" Really? Seriously?? No. The government approved its use for chemo patients, and any company that wouldn't hire you because you used pot to help curb nausea while being treated for cancer...well, is that the kind of company you'd even want to work for? Say it with me, "HellNoInaHandBasket."

It took me a while to relax on this subject, so I get it if you're unsure. One thing about this unfamiliar road you're walking on, is that you're going to see, feel, and experience things you may have never thought about. You are going to see life from a whole different perspective. I was going to say your vision would go from myopic to something that sounded broad, but that doesn't quite cut it. It's more like it shatters your image of life into nearly unrecognizable pieces and scatters it all around, then a gust of wind comes along and blows it all away. It's all very *The Matrix*. It's a little scary at first, but it's very freeing to no longer be afraid of death. You'll experience life on a much deeper level now, than you did before. A level where you don't really care what the neighbors might think.

Mary Jane and her buddies; the anti-anxiety meds and other symptom relievers you'll be offered are all being offered for a reason; to help you get to a place where you are calm and your primary focus is on the fight. Don't be afraid to reach out and take a chill pill when natural methods just aren't enough.

So, now that you've got a super cool, laid-back friend, it's time to acquire a new phobia...

CHAPTER 9
GERMAPHOBES "R" US

🚲 🚲 🚲

All that talk about how you need to chill out and relax, and now I say, what? Okay, I don't mean you need to go to the extreme like Howie Mandel, who (poor guy) thinks the palm of his hand is like a petri dish. Leave OCD to the professionals. You need, however, to become acutely aware of the germs around you and how to stay clear of them whenever possible. Remember the "5 second rule?' Well, replace that with "You drop it, you toss it."

The first time this really hit home was at chemo, when I was taking notes and without thinking I put the pen in my mouth, to free both of my hands for typing. Rachel, one of the nurses, nearly shouted at me from across the room, "Ali, nooooooo! Get that out of your mouth!" You'd think I was about to pull the pin out of a grenade, the way she came at me. FYI, I read this to Rachel, and she considers this an over dramatization, but she agrees with the strength of my recommendation to keep germy items out of your mouth.

Let me add, you should definitely keep these things out of your eyes as well. Conjunctivitis (pink eye) sucks anytime, but it's ten times worse when you're slow to heal. While you're on chemo my friend, you are definitely slow to heal. I also wear contacts, and at the time, refused to invest in a pair of prescription glasses because I'm stupidly vain sometimes. It was allergy season, so I kept rubbing my eyes with my germy fingers…under protected windows to the soul/body…need I say more?

Here are some examples of ways we expose ourselves to germs everyday without thinking; pumping gas, riding an escalator, handling door knobs, holding cell phones, touching railings as you go up and down stairs, picking up fruits and vegetables in the market, computer keyboards, wearing a bra too long, unsterilized toothbrush, slobbery pet kisses, drinking from a can, using card readers at stores, ATM machines, and handling money, for starters...

You don't need to stop doing all of these things, or walk around in a hazmat suit, but there are a few simple precautions you should take. First, get a few of those little bottles of anti-bacterial gel (most drug stores sell them). Put one in your bathroom, purse, coat pocket, desk, wherever you'd come in contact with potentially dangerous germs. You should have it with you at all times, and use it just after coming in contact. Don't drink out of the same cup as others, or share silverware when dining. I know, simple pleasures, but not so simple when your white blood cell count is bottoming out.

Another way to protect yourself is to send an update to your friends once chemo starts, letting them in on your new food and beverage prep needs. People will want to cook for you, and you should let them, trust me. Gently inform them of your new germ warfare. Believe me, many don't make the connection, that they need to stay clear if they've been exposed to anything contagious. This is true even of something seemingly nonthreatening, such as the common cold. My big mistake was not washing my hands after petting my friend's dogs. I'm slightly allergic to pet dander, but they're a hypoallergenic breed, so now worries right? They go outside all the time. They roll around on the grass, sidewalks, streets and yes, they are full of germs as my red gooey eyes could attest. It took a full week for them to clear, and I was rinsing them constantly, with every remedy I could get my hands on. It's your turn to be selfish and incredibly self-protective. And yes, they probably would have healed faster if I just had those spare glasses... I have them now, by the way. Can't nobody say I don't never evolve.

Okay, where else...ehm, seemingly harmless places such as; pubs, restaurants, and even outdoor events can be hazardous terrain. The wind blows all kinds of germy things about. Bars and restaurants try to keep things clean, but how many times have you sat at a table, and noticed they missed a few spots with their cold, wet rag? We shrug or turn a blind eye when we're strong because we know we can fight off those little wimpy germs. Well, now you're the little wimp, they're finally bigger and badder than you, and they're chomping at the bit to prove it. Don't give them the chance. The road you're on is rough enough without having to add an infection to the pile.

Other things to avoid (this is tough when your treatment moves through the holidays, and other favorite events), are airplanes, trains and busses. They are the worst of the worst, with all that recycled air, and if you think they wipe down all the seat arms and tray tables with antibacterial cleanser, then congratulations your new name is Pollyanna. It was my name when I decided to go against Dr. H.'s advice, and go home for Thanksgiving one year. This was just barely two months into chemo. I figured I wasn't that far into it yet and my white blood cell count (WBC) was just over the danger line, before you have to endure the dreaded booster shot.

Additionally, I hadn't seen my family since I broke the news, and I felt a strong pull to see them, to have them see me, which I knew would put their minds at ease. Plus, my sister puts on an amazing Thanksgiving feast every year, and I hated to miss it. I was still glad I went, but it came at a price.

Just after I got back it became painful to pee, and there was a tiny bit of blood in my urine, which they immediately tested, and found I had a urinary tract infection. Ouch. It could've meant postponement of treatment, but it was an off week. There are different schedules for treatment. Mine, was alternating one week on and one week off. To remedy the UTI, I went on antibiotics for a week, bought the local grocer out of cranberry juice, and swore never to ignore Dr. H.'s advice again.

Have I freaked you out yet? I hope not. There's no need to freak. You just need to see all this stuff with a new set of protective eyes, so you can avoid these obstacles to the success of your treatment and recovery. Wash all your fresh vegetables and fruits before eating them, and keep a little bottle of that antibacterial stuff with you at all times, so you can wipe your hands wherever and whenever. When you're at a restaurant, go for the cooked stuff and for fkssake stop sharing forks, glasses, and the like, with your loved ones. It's sweet. It's endearing, and it's just asking for trouble. Just think how much sweeter it will be when you're all done with treatment, healthy enough to handle it, and headed into your new lease on life. Some things are genuinely worth waiting for.

With all this hand washing and sanitizing, you can guess what else you need to stock up on; moisturizer, and get the good stuff. I actually used Neosporin for my fingertips because they seemed to get the worst of it. To each their own brand, but I like the moisturizers that smell like things I love. For example; I bought salt scrub that smelled like fresh grapefruit, and another that smelled like lemon. I also bought body cream that smelled like blueberries (Yummm). I put a little on my upper lip, especially when the chemical taste/smell invaded my sinuses. It was a nice, little momentary reprieve.

Oh, they'll probably tell you this, but it bears mentioning here. They warned me to avoid manicures and pedicures. I didn't get it at first, but when you think about it, they often use sharp instruments that bore into the skin, and expose it to all kinds of germs. All shops claim to be clean (and to the average eye they seem it), but they say it's not worth the risk. I had a regular manicurist because I'm useless at doing it myself and I always end up with nail polish all over the place. I warned her of the risks and she went into extra gentle mode with me, but again, ask your doc beforehand. They're the experts on your safety and well being, right now.

While it's important to play it safe, pampering yourself is also really important. Whether you're a man, woman or child, find whatever makes you happy. Maybe it's massage therapy, hydro therapy or shopping therapy. If it is OK'd by the boss of you, go for it every chance you can get. Just stay away from steam sauna/jacuzzi…it sounds good, but it's a germ fest in there.

I know, you're right. We should cover this, "But Ali, what is a normal WBC level and when is it dangerous?" 4.0-10 is normal and 1.0 means you're getting the dreaded "booster shot." I've been there a couple times, but not since I started adding all the supplements to my daily routine. The lowest my WBC dropped to was 1.2, so bear that in mind when you think of skipping out on those extra steps.

Well, now look at you…you've got all your questions answered, you are incredibly fearless, all your loved ones are in the know and clear on giving you what you need, your house and head are clean as a whistle, your medicine cabinet is filled to the brim, you've made a new super laid-back friend, and you've got all you need to become a bona fide Germaphobe. Now, it's time to go *au naturel*…

CHAPTER 10
NUTURE WITH NATURE –
NUTRITION TIPS

🚲 🚲 🚲

Since eating healthy and maintaining a healthy weight has been my biggest struggle, I decided to bring in an expert on the subject, for guidance on my; "Nuture with Nature" mantra.

Mary Hollander, RN/RMT, was the nutrition counselor at the cancer center, when I first arrived. She offers classes and sends regular, informative nutrition updates to all us cancer fighters. She also hosts some really informative nutrition blogs. Reading these always cheers me up and makes me feel just a little bit smarter and more powerful. You know what they say about knowledge and power...I posed the top nutrition Q's to Mary and here's what she came back with...

"During chemotherapy and/or radiation therapy, maintaining a healthy immune system should be your goal. Diet, exercise, and stress management can help you attain this.

Because you are an individual, not a statistic, your cancer experience will be different from anyone else's. Keeping a food diary will be very important. Write down the foods you eat each day. Add how you felt physically, emotionally, and if you had any symptoms such as diarrhea, nausea, or pain. When you experience the same side effect the next day or week, go back and compare the foods you have eaten. This will help you build a list of foods that work for you, and which to avoid.

Here are a few tips to help you during treatment. Pick what works for you."

CHANGES IN TASTE AND SMELL
A metallic taste is the most common.

Avoid: Red meat & food with strong odors. Any foods that are unappealing to you at this time.

Eat: Add flavor to your food with spices. Broiled or baked mild flavored meats: chicken turkey & fish. Try flavoring your water with lemon, cucumber and/or mint.

Tips: Use plastic or wooden utensils; glass or ceramic cooking pots. Avoid metal utensils, canned foods, and metal pots & pans.

CONSTIPATION

Avoid: Processed foods, white foods (rice bread and pasta), red meat & dairy.

Eat: High fiber foods, such as whole grains, beans, nut butters, vegetables (the lowly radish is very high in fiber & a natural detox food) & fruits. A fresh, whole pear, kiwi or prunes, eaten an hour before breakfast, will keep you regular. A glass of warm water with lemon juice first thing every morning, helps to keep you moving as well.

Tip: Keeping yourself hydrated is very important. Fiber requires fluids. Herbal teas such as *Smooth Move* by Traditional Medicinals & *Get Regular* by Yogi Tea are safe to use. Have one cup each evening.

DIARRHEA

Avoid: Sugary drinks including fruit juices, greasy & fried foods, dairy, alcohol & spicy foods.

Eat: Eat potassium and sodium rich foods such as miso soup, bananas, peaches & white potatoes. Low fiber foods are needed in this case: white rice, pasta, low fiber bread, cream of wheat, baked or broiled lean meats.

Tip: Have all foods at room temperature. Increase your water intake to replace the fluids you lose. Chamomile, ginger or mint tea will help settle the stomach.

LOSS OF APPETITE

Avoid: Processed foods, added sugar, sodas & foods with strong odors.

Eat: High calorie, nutrient dense snacks. Nut butter on whole grain bread or crackers, small portion of turkey, chicken or fish, avocado, whole fruits (fruit juice is too high in sugar without the fiber), hummus, oatmeal, nuts & seeds.

Tip: Eating small meals and grab & go snacks frequently, during the day, will work better than the traditional 3 meals. By eating 6 to 8 snacks/meals a day, you will take in more calories. Ginger chews or tea, 2-3 times a day, will stimulate your appetite. A drop of orange oil on your napkin will also stimulate your appetite!

MOUTH SORES

Avoid: Spicy foods, alcohol, acidic foods, rough, course or dry foods

Eat: Soft foods, mashed yams/potatoes, smoothies, oatmeal, bananas & applesauce. Pureed fruits, vegetables & meats, if the sores are causing difficulty with swallowing.

Tip: Eating a tablespoon of dark honey, slowly (Manuka honey is very beneficial), will not only coat your mouth and throat, it will promote healing. Sip water frequently, keeping your mouth moist. Rinse your mouth with salt water after each meal.

NAUSEA

Avoid: Strong odors, greasy & fried foods, sugar laden drinks & foods.

Eat: Warm cereals, soups & low fat protein foods; skinned chicken & tempeh, for example. Ginger chews or crystallized ginger helps with all types of nausea.

Tip: Small meals or snacks. Hydrate! Being dehydrated can cause nausea & headaches. Drinking mint or ginger teas during the day also relieves nausea. Keep crackers at your bedside or in your purse, along with the ginger chews.

THRUSH
An oral yeast infection caused by candida albicans.

Avoid: Sugar (all types) and yeast-containing foods. Foods such as bread, beer and wine, encourage candida growth. Avoid sprouted whole grains. Kambucha is popular, but should also be avoided in cases of thrush. Dairy; butter milk, cheese & yogurt.

Eat: Garlic 1 clove raw, if tolerated, per day. Eggs, avocado, nuts & seeds. Eat lean meat; chicken, turkey & fish. Fruits, vegetables, beans, whole grains and spices (if they don't irritate your mouth).

Tip: Plain yogurt (the exception) with lactobacillus acidophilus (in small amounts), will act as a probiotic. It will keep your 'gut buddies' healthy. An alternative to the yogurt is to take a dairy free probiotic daily. If you are having difficulty swallowing, consider pureeing your meals.

Isn't Mary awesome? I wasn't sure why she recommended "warm or hot" water, so I ask her, and I learned a new thing. Warm (almost hot) water stimulates the digestive system to work. She also told me a really interesting story. "When I was a young nurse, an older surgeon wrote that as an order for all his surgical patients, starting the morning after surgery. His patients were the only ones who pooped & peed right after surgery, allowing them a shorter hospital stay! The ones on meds had a difficult recovery." If you're ever in surgery again, or the trains are slow-going, drink hot water with lemon. The things I learn~

CHAPTER 11
DRINK LIKE A FISH, SWEAT LIKE A PIG, AND PEE LIKE A RUSSIAN RACE HORSE

☙ ☙ ☙

Yup, it's pretty much that simple. You need to hydrate. You need to sweat, and you need to pee out those toxins. With so much of our bodies being made up of water, what's with the big push to drink at least a half-gallon of it every day? You'll actually notice it yourself if you don't follow this recommendation. I didn't. In fact, I stubbornly refused (Ohhh, why must I always learn the hard way?) to take heed. You'll suddenly notice the back scratchers (two at a time) as you wait in line at the pharmacy, and want to grab them off the rack and use them, right then and there. Your hands and the skin around your feet and ankles will feel tight from the dryness, and then a light bulb will go off in your head...

There are two kinds of hydration you need. The first is in your hands, as in, you should be holding a bottle or tall glass of water right now. You're not? How 'bout you go do that now. It's ok, I'll wait. It's totally cool. I don't mind...

Some people buy it by the bottle, or have it delivered. If I could go back, I'd have it delivered. It seems such an easy reminder to fill up on water when you know a truck is coming to take the bottle away and replace it with another one. I fought this hydration thing tooth and nail because I'm almost never thirsty (unless a margarita is placed before me). I felt as if I was forcing water down as a kind of punishment or something. I had the best intentions, and bought a bunch of those reusable water bottles, but then I got wigged out over the germiness of them.

After that, I went for the twelve-pack of 32 oz bottles, and added fresh lemon lime or unsweetened cranberry juice, and pretended I was being très chic about it all. I kept a bottle on the bathroom counter to drink down the meds throughout the day and one by my chair, where I'd watch TV (my favorite escape) at night. That seemed to do the trick. Also, the fear of another urinary tract infection helped keep me in line.

Since then, that large bottle of cranberry water is far more appealing. After four years of constant use, I am a firm believer in drinking alkaline water. Look it up. It's considered to be really good for detoxing your body. We have a massive supply in the town over, so I just go there once a week, rinse and refill my three-gallon jug, plus a gallon jug I keep in the bathroom to swallow down all those morning pills. It's very European, so, of course, we (Americans who crave ties to our European heritage) are all into it.

The second type of hydration is; cellular. No, not the kind of cellular you ring up your friends on. It's the kind that is teeny-tiny, and fighting off those cancer cells. When you hydrate at the cellular level, you're making a big move in flushing those excess chemicals, that have been pumped into your body, out of your system. You don't want them piling up in there, trust me. Drinking water helps flush the toxins out too, so imagine how much faster you'll recover when you go for both. How does cellular hydration happen? Your nurse will ask you if you want it at the end of your chemo cycle and usually you'll get it during, via an IV bag. Again, every schedule is different, but after chemo they'd offer to follow it up with hydration before I headed home. The following week I'd come in for a blood draw (because they like to keep close tabs on your white blood cell count and be sure there are no infections going on in there), and they'd ask if I wanted to stay for hydration. I said, "No thanks," most of the time, and I'd be on my merry way, until I realized how much easier it would be to recover from a chemo cycle if I just said, "Yes," to it. If they don't offer, ask for it on every cycle.

I know, "Sweat like a pig" isn't the nicest term, and it conjures up images that seem rather unpleasant, but this is just as important as the hydration mantra we've taken on. I'm living proof of how much longer it sucks, when you don't get up, and get active after your chemo cycle. Just imagine, all that water you're sucking down, that they've pumped into your body... it's sloshing around inside you with all those chemicals. How are you going to push all that out? Thanks to salt intake and edema (swelling) caused by treatment, it's not going to pass out of your body as easily as before, so you need to give it a little push and they say sweating it out is the second best way to do it (peeing is #1).

Walking with someone worked well for me, or hopping on my bike for a half hour or more. Best of all, was swimming, but only when your WBC is at a good level. If mine was 3.0 or higher then I went for it. One hour in the pool, with my little floaties and snorkel gear, and I swear I'd pee out 5 lbs. Some days I could barely stand, I was so tired, so I lay on a mat, used a stretch band and stretched my legs and arms. Even that little bit can make a difference. Just be sure whatever you do, it's OK'd by your doc, and if you're straying from home (traveling or the gym), make sure you have a workout buddy, in case it becomes too much to handle. Try to go right after you get unplugged from chemo. The sooner you get your body moving, the sooner that crap gets out of your body, and you will start to feel better. People ask me if the cancer makes me sick. I say, "No, I don't even feel the cancer. It's the chemo that knocks me on my butt."

The goal is to sweat from head to toe. The hair on the back of your neck should be dripping wet, when you're done. Be sure to stretch before and after and…you guessed it: HYDRATE. Take at least a 32 oz bottle of water with you to the gym or your workout area at home and it should be empty by the time you finish your workout.

It's important to remember that even if you've gained considerable weight during treatment this is not a "weight" thing. This is a, "flush those toxins from my body," thing.

That said, don't push. Just don't waste that energy with a, "Hey everyone, I feel great. Let's go out and eat, drink and be merry tonight." I did that in the beginning because I was so determined to show my friends how tough/un-phased I was. Each time I did, I woke up the next day feeling sick as a dog and flu-ish. I never said I was the smartest bird in the tree. When they told me I needed to do another three months of maintenance chemo, I saw it as a second chance to get it right. I've definitely stuck to my own exercise advice more this time, but it's a constant struggle because a: I hate exercising, and my brain isn't good at being consistent at anything. I'm from a long line of couch potatoes, who talk far more about what's for dinner, than what's the best workout. Ah, well it's never too late to change, evolve, and break the chains that bind us to the past. Never say Never~

I know what you're thinking, "But Ali, how will I know if I'm hydrating enough or not?" Good question Look at you, coming up with all the right questions~ And, here's where we're going to talk about pee. Yes, the mantra, "Pee like a Russian racehorse," is a good one, and it's important to pay attention to the color of your pee each time you go because it can tell you if you're drinking enough liquids or not (or worse, if a urinary tract infection is coming on).

Okay, here's the gamut by colors: Clear = You are drinking waaaay too much water. Cut back. Light yellow = Good job. You are hydrating just the right amount. If it's slightly darker yellow, it's still considered a "normal" level, but your next stop should be for a glass of water. Any darker and you are definitely dehydrated. If there is any pink in it (that's probably blood), that could be a sign of urinary tract infection. Don't freak out, just call your doctor during office hours and let them know. They'll sort it out. The important thing is not to let it go unspoken or untreated. "Stay on top of the side effects." That's what Chris, the P.A. told me when I first started, and he was absolutely right. When I do, it's so much easier to handle chemo, than when I don't.

Though this wasn't in the title of the chapter it is an important factor in detoxing...one of my best friends likes to refer to it as "the trains." As in, "The trains are running well today." Or, "The trains have yet to leave the station." How do you know how often "the trains" should run? One of my favorite health experts (and former film heart throb), Frank Jasper, said it best, and basically, "Every 24 hours." So, if you haven't gone (#2) in more than 24 hours, then you need to reach into the medicine cabinet and get out the laxatives/prompters, whatever works best for you. Frank goes into more detail on *The C Card and Me* website, but that's the gist. Chemo is extremely dehydrating and I'm just going to say it, "There's nothing worse than being stuffed full of toxic poo." There you go, I said it. You are now officially informed and forewarned.

Well, there you. You've got all your questions answered, you are obstinately fearless, you've got all your loved ones in the know, and waiting on you hand and foot, your house and head are spick-and-span, your medicine cabinet is bustin' out, you've made a new super laid-back friend, you've got all you need to become a bona fide germaphobe, and you slosh as you walk you're so full of water. Even better, you have all the know-how on flushing this crap out of your system between cycles. Are you feeling nice and full from this bounty of knowledge? Well, pat dat belly and settle in, 'cuz it's time to do a little daydreaming...

CHAPTER 12
DO WHAT YOU LOVE, AND THE
HEALING WILL FOLLOW

🚲 🚲 🚲

I'll bet you have started thinking about and possibly lamenting all the things you wanted to do in life and thought you had all the time in the world to do. Now you've started to wonder if you'll ever get the chance. This is another part of your whole new perception or outlook on life. That worry dissipates and soon you'll start mapping out how and when to make one of those things on your bucket list happen. This is important. You need to have something to look forward to when the treatment is over and you need to be able to visualize it. Imagine how you'll board that plane, get off at your long-awaited destination, and enjoy the trip all the more than you would've before when you were just taking life for granted or trudging your way through.

Even with all the financial help, I did have to put a lot of my dreams on the back burner. This included recording a full-length CD, which is what I was in the midst of planning when the bad news broke. It also included holding off on long vacations with friends to Europe and Mexico. I dreamed of going to Isla Mujeres the whole first year of treatment. I was going to take half my tax return and set it aside for that. I was supposed to be finished with chemo (or so I thought) in the spring. I was going to give it two months for the sensitivity to sunlight to wear off and then off I'd go to stroll the beaches, down some margaritas at the local cantina with my friends, and brave another fear by swimming with sharks. They'd be nurse sharks, of course, not the bitey kind. I am braver these days, but I'm not quite that brave (or crazy) yet. Not one to give up, I readjusted my vision of how and when these things would happen. Being cash poor has been a great lesson in frugality (ugh) and how to be far more clever about money. Other things come first, and they may sidetrack your dates or the degree to which you'll afford to make that dream happen, but you should always have something to look forward to. Make a list of all the things you'd like to do and places you'd like to go, and start planning for them. Decide who you'd like to go with and get them involved. Planning is half the fun you know, and it's a great way to take your minds off darker matters.

Those words you just read...I wrote them three years ago. As I'm reading them over again I'm busting out in a big smile because since I wrote them I have been to Ireland (twice) Italy (twice) and been to Isla Mujeres Mexico. It wasn't whale shark season, but I had a great time with friends and made new ones, just as I imagined I would.

At one point on the trip, I was faced with an opportunity to sit in a little water pen with nurse sharks (about 3 feet long), but I hesitated. A handsome man with a Greek accent stopped and asked me if I was going in. I suggested he go first to make sure they were safe (yes, this was my sad attempt at flirting). He said he'd already gone in, and asked me if I was hesitating because I was afraid or because I didn't like the idea of it. I answered, "Both, but mostly I'm afraid." He smiled warmly, and said (in that beautifully vibrant way that the Greeks express themselves), "You must face your fears!" I told him I'd consider it, as he headed off to his party boat.

I decided in the end, that I disliked the idea of penning up these creatures and letting droves of strangers pet them daily for a few pesos more than I feared going into the pen, but to pay respect to my handsome messenger, the next day I signed up for an open sea snorkeling adventure. Twice I dove into the sea with a small group of fellow tourists and our guide. Only once did I panic; when I looked up from the water to see they were all pretty far from me, and I was even farther from the boat. I impulsively doggie paddled for a few seconds before realizing how ridiculous that looked even if I were to be bitten by a shark. No witness would ever be able to tell the tale with a straight face, so I dropped my mask covered face back in the water and pumped my fins with all my might, until I made it safely back on board the boat.

Among other post daunting-diagnosis accomplishments; I recorded that full length CD of my original music (entitled *Piece of Cake*), and launched it on iTunes. We even had a fancy launch party to mark the occasion. There was a memorable sisters' trip to New York, to see my niece, meet cousins for the first time, and re-unite with some of my favorite people on the planet. I am always amazed when I see someone again in a different time and place than when and where I got to know them. In that moment, you realize you could change out the scenery and time period like clothes on a paper doll, but the indescribable thing that makes you resonate together remains intact. Man, I love those moments, and that's quite a few checks off the bucket list~ All within a three year span, and many done right in-between chemo cycles, giving just an extra week in-between. Of course, those were contingent on my WBC being high enough and Dr. H.'s (albeit, sometimes reluctant) approval.

Ok, your turn. Get a pen and write it down here and now. Go on, it'll feel good. Write your top three things you'd like to do before you kick the bucket. Write down; what, where, who and when. Include a ballpark figure of what you think it'll cost. That may help you decide which order to go after them.

THINGS TO LOOK FORWARD TO

What:

Where:

With Whom:

When:

How Much-ish:

What:

Where:

With Whom:

When: How Much-ish:

What:

Where:

With Whom:

When:

How Much-ish:

Hold onto those wishes and make them known to anyone who'll hear them. It's really fun to plan these trips out with whomever you want to go with, and it'll be a great break from your new routine. One of the great things (look, another silver lining) about going on medical leave (besides the much needed rest) is you'll have far more time than you'll know what to do with. I slept a lot and caught up on a lot of movies, but it also gave me time to work on my music, songwriting and photography.

I also did some in-depth planning on how to ease back into the work world with my newfound, far more creative skills. Of course, that was my denial in thinking chemo brain wouldn't affect my sense of memory, or ability to learn new things. I still keep at it daily, stimulating the brain every chance I can get and working on getting my body and mind to the strongest place they can be. At times, it makes me feel emotional. Whether the emotion is; sadness, relief, anger, or frustration, it surfaces whenever I hit a roadblock from my previous abilities/super-powers. However, I am grateful to the fantastic brains that have been instrumental in deciphering the words I spit out onto paper, helping them all make much more sense to you, the reader, so let's all say it together, "Thank you Micheeeelle~"

If this virtual c card brings you anything, I hope it acts as a constant reminder that you have earned the right to make it all about you right now. It truly is your turn to be selfish, regardless of what anyone says or does. It's going to be really difficult for those of you raised to put all others first. Parents, especially, will find this hard, but you must. There's no point in investing all this time money and energy into your treatment if you're not going to put yourself first. The docs and nurses can't do it all. You have to put your oar in as well and start paddling. If it helps, think of it this way; when you're on an airplane, and the flight attendant goes over the safety procedures, they tell you to put the oxygen mask on yourself first because if you take care of you first then you'll be able to take care of others.

Part of putting yourself first, means unapologetically choosing which social agendas to keep up with and which ones to drop for now (or for good). You can and should still do a lot of the things you enjoy in life. You just need to re-portion these activities to fit within your new schedule and energy reserve. Singing is definitely something I love to do. The week of chemo and the few days surrounding it though I couldn't. One of the side effects of my treatment was locked-up vocal cords, which made my throat feel kind of sore/tight, and my voice sounded like it had a constant frogginess to it. Then, add in the post-nasal drip. Oh, how I HATE most of the side effects. You're sitting there talking to someone, and then suddenly, you're dripping away, while frantically searching your purse for something to sop it up.

This road ain't pretty. There are a lot of little embarrassing moments heading your way. Just take them in stride, and let yourself (and others) laugh through them when they happen. Be sure to surround yourself with people who can find the humor in it all. Humor is one of the mightiest of endorphin builders.

Remember, with chemo brain you probably won't be able to handle intricate things. Your brain will just skip a beat here and there and you'll find yourself lost in the middle of expressing a thought. I've actually blanked completely on new friends' names. The heart stays intact though. I would beam at the site of them, but their names were just nowhere to be found. One friend's favorite moment was when I would space out while someone was talking to me and then moments later I would repeat what that person said as if it was my idea, only I couldn't remember how I got that idea. They try not to show their frustration, but you know it's there. Of course, it's there.

I'd highly recommend getting really comfortable with your phone's calendar feature. It's a great tool for managing all the (now difficult to remember) appointment dates and times. If you have an old dinosaur of a phone, upgrade now. If possible, get a similar type. Nothing is worse than learning new technology while all this is going on. I did, and I've worked in technology for over fifteen years. It didn't matter.

With chemo brain, I felt like a primate trying to figure out the mysterious black shiny thing. I used the calendar on my phone to remind me where I needed to be every day and when. I also used it to write notes to myself when I came up with an idea, or an errand that needed to be carried out later. I'd sometimes forget details as I was typing in into the phone. It's the strangest feeling. I chose to make light of it. Most people went along and when they didn't...I whipped out my c card, as if to say, "Give me a fekkn break, would ya? I'd like to see how well you'd do in this situation."

When it comes to this part of the guide, I don't think you need to write out your favorite things to do. Let it just come to you and decide on the spot if you want to do something or not. Do NOT be afraid to disappoint others by canceling the day of or even an hour before. Your mood and energy levels will fluctuate without much notice. Learn to listen to your body and give it precedence.

That was a hard one to learn for me. I hated missing out on all the fun and catching up. I'd get dressed up and mid-way through getting ready I'd start sweating. Then I'd look in the mirror and I'd see this pasty gray bloated face staring back at me. I looked like something on a morgue slab. I'd pout, then cry my eyes out for a bit while texting my cancellation, and then I'd shake it off, change into my super soft PJs, pour myself a big glass of bitter cranberry water, put on a funny movie, and all was right-ish with the world again. Always trust your instincts and listen your body.

How 'bout this for a recap...when you opened this book your head was still reeling from the news. Now, you've got all your questions answered, you are brilliantly fearless, all your loved ones are in the know and clear on giving you what you need, your house and head are clean as a whistle, your medicine cabinet is filled to the brim, you've made a new super laid-back friend, you've got all you need to become a bonafide germaphobe, and you're a veritable irrigation system. Even better, you have all the know-how on flushing this stuff out of your system between cycles.

You've got some insider info on the money part of it. That should start to put your mind at ease if that's a stressor, and if not, you've been given some ideas on how to increase your health-improving endorphins, while helping take the burden off of others. You've got at least three things to look forward to after the treatment is complete, and you can continue to do what you love (just in smaller doses). Feel free to explore new things that fit within your new schedule and fluctuating energy levels. Keep in the forefront of your mind at all times...YOU.

Never forget the importance of endorphins and what brings them on: exercising, laughing, smiling, flirting, hugging, being around people whose company you enjoy, doing social things you love, trying new things, giving yourself things to look forward to when it's over and planning for them.

You've got a medicine cabinet that's chock-full and don't you be afraid to use it. Stay on top of those symptoms. That's the trick. Take something the moment those symptoms come on. Once again, there are no guarantees for anyone on the outcome, but the road will definitely be much smoother for you if you follow these suggestions.

Even with all these pluses in your pocket, there will be "those" moments, "those" days. Time to reach into the expert input reserve for this one...

CHAPTER 13
I'M GIVING HER ALL SHE'S GOT CAPTAIN (HOW TO COPE WHEN YOU FEEL YOU'VE REACHED YOUR LIMIT)

🚲 🚲 🚲

Last summer, when I was clearing out my mother's sewing room, I found this framed quote on the desk. It said, "The discipline of a writer is to learn to be still and listen to what his subject has to tell him." It reminded me of some feedback I'd received on the book, "I hope she plans to expand her book and flesh things out a bit more." Another reader said, "With a recent metastatic cancer diagnosis, I was looking for information and coping hints." Those two have been rolling around in my head since I first read them. They were actually a huge part of my decision to write the second book, and expand the website/blogs.

Since I'm not a bonafide expert on coping skills, and this is an area that readers asked for more depth on, I turned to therapist Eve Beutler, MFT, Founder of Cancer Angels of San Diego. I asked for her input on how to cope with the downside of cancer and here's what she had to say:

Dealing with the depression, stress, and sense of hopelessness that often comes with waking up to cancer each day, requires the cancer warrior to give value not only to life, but to her/his every moment. Any value that you have given yourself based primarily on your physical capabilities, your looks, your income, your work, what you do (e.g., a CEO...a teacher...a full-time mom), must take a second seat to first valuing and fighting for the core person you are. Let that sink in for a moment.

You must re-define yourself each day when battling a chronic disease. Yes, a chronic, not incurable or terminal illness. Having dealt with a lung disease since the age of 8, given countless death sentences, I promise you; a day alive is a day in the time bank. I was completely certain that my days were numbered, that my husband was looking for a replacement, that my kids had accepted the awful progression of the lung disease, when seemingly out of nowhere a new drug was discovered to treat the rare lung disease with which I live fully every day. I had to hold on for FDA approval, which can take what feels like forever. Now, here I am telling you there are hundreds of clinical trials and hundreds of off label drugs either on the market or coming to the market, which will destroy or at least put at bay the monster...the "C" word.

To simply face each day, even when you are feeling terrible, here are some of the things to which you must wholeheartedly commit. These are body, soul, mind, and heart commitments.

TAKE TIME FOR YOURSELF WITHOUT DISTRACTIONS

Research shows, that allowing yourself to achieve a higher state, be it through prayer, meditation, yoga, music -- whatever allows you to completely clear your mind and be in the moment (sounds easier than it is, but it happens with practice), increases the T cells that fight the cancer cells. This practice of achieving a higher state, using more than 10% of your brain, should be implemented each day.

MAKE YOURSELF A SACRED CONTAINER OF PRECIOUS DAYS

How about putting something in a sacred container for every day of just living? It's your savings account of time buying. Throw it in hard if you need to…let the frustration go right in with it. You will be amazed when you see that you need a second container, and a third. You will remember how hopeless you might have felt in the beginning, and now how hopeful you should feel…you are still alive and not giving in. Just allowing yourself to ride the swings of ups and downs is an accomplishment. Give yourself acknowledgment for that. No one, but you, can understand what it feels like to be in your situation. Tune out those that think they do and offer unsolicited advice.

VALUE YOURSELF

When your body feels terrible, when your mind screams, "Get up you lazy person," and you can't move without vomiting or being in pain, LOVE YOUR BODY. Stop being angry at your body for turning on you. It hasn't. I rejected my lungs for about 30 years, until I realized I had to love and nurture them. They were struggling to breathe. They were pushing hard while I was working against them. I needed to slow down, visualize them in cool aqua waters floating (that's my vision…you pick yours), and do what they asked of me. Usually, they said, "Please slow down. Please redefine yourself." It's ok if you're not the same as you used to be. You are a new you and we need to work together. Please listen. Fighting your body, listening to "should's," listening to external chatter from just about every one telling you about alternative cures, toxins, what you need to do to cure yourself...tell them to "Back off." Your body, your temporary you, needs to feel worthwhile.

When you feel sick, be sick. Isolate. When you feel well, share a little bit of wisdom about the importance of living and not taking things for granted. Now, you know how lucky one is just to have health! Know you are valuable. Even though your body is different, your soul is the same...maybe becoming even better...maybe growing...even inspiring someone around you.

GIVE IN TO YOUR DESIRES FOR A FULL DAY

Since it's a daily journey, have a "Fuggid all" day. Let yourself have a mini-breakdown. Cry. Scream. Cuss out the unfairness. Watch a movie and cry some more or laugh. Eat whatever the heck you want. It's not going to kill you. You may not feel great the next day, but so what? Feel good today. Don't talk to anyone. Make no commitments. Just let it all hang out. Wake up the next day and see if you're ready to start fighting again. Find someone with whom you can share some laughter or an ice cream sundae...whatever you want. Call a friend and say, "I'm having a fuggid all day, want to join me?"

GET CLARITY

Write down all of the reasons you are depressed on a sheet of paper. Divide this sheet into three columns. The columns are, "I have control. I have some control. I have no control." Look at each column, do the necessary things over which you have control and let go of worrying about those things over which you have none. We've all heard that old saying, but doing it is more complicated because you really have to think about it. There will be things you thought you had control over, that you don't and vice versa. You may even find that you don't know which issue fits where in your "control" columns. Once you do, let go. Worry has NO value and can harm you. The definition of worry is, "To torment oneself with or suffer from disturbing thoughts." Why in the world would anyone do that? Make sure you stop any negative spiraling, no matter what it takes.

NEGATIVE SPIRALING

Identify when you are going into a negative spiral. A negative spiral takes a simple, bad day and turns it into, "I might as well give up. I'm going to suffer and die. I can't get out of bed." This spiral can be identified by first accepting what your body is feeling. Address it. Is there anything you can do to make it feel better? Do you need rest? Food? Companionship? Distraction? Music? Pain killer? What do you need to restart, to let go of the thoughts and start over? Often, just going to sleep for a while or forcing yourself to take a walk around the block, if possible, can stop the spiral. The hardest thing may be to reach out to someone. Learn to do this. Reach out to a friend or family member. Develop a code for friends to know you are spiraling, so you don't have to say it...like, "Code green," could mean, "I'm lonely." "Code red," could mean you feel so angry about everything that you just can't function. Come up with ways to communicate the panic or depression that begins the negative spiral. Give yourself time to process test results, chemo, radiation...then reach out. Identify in your body what it feels like when the negative spiral is about to grab you. You will begin to recognize this and become proactive. It is a feeling that may start in your chest or in your head, but once identified you can nip it in the bud.

BE IN THE NOW, BUT NOT REALLY, NOT FOR LONG, BUT ONLY NOW, BUT...

It's very confusing to be told to take each moment at a time when that particular moment feels unbearable. If you stay in it, you can feel hopeless like giving up. If you try to leave it, you feel helpless and unable to fight your body. How do you know when you should, "listen to your body" versus "make a run for it?" Focus on the next moments; remember the times when you feel good, remember that it's temporary...without getting into an all out war with your body.

It's so easy to forget feeling good. It's easy to forget just how long it took you to get through the last chemo cycle, the last bad news, the last overwhelming block of pain. If you can't remember how long it took you, if you can only feel the current distress, how do you get out of the misery of the moment?

Learn a body shorthand. Get yourself a little journal and put notes in it to remind you of the drill. For example: Tuesday -- chemo 1-5. Went home, rested, ate, fell asleep. Wednesday -- woke up feeling a little tired, but no big deal. Thursday -- I feel like I want to die. Nauseous. Vomiting. Weak. Headache. Pain. Going to bed. Friday -- still run over by truck, drank some soup. Saturday -- body aches gone.

Keeping this short, but consistent, journal will remind you that you made it through the last round, the last "test," the last "challenge." Even though it feels like you'll never get through it, you can read it right there. These are our reality reminders that we can get through this extremely tough time.

Once you know what your body is asking, allow yourself to rest and sleep. Set an alarm clock to wake you up if you're going to sleep due to depression versus true physical illness. Sometimes, it's hard to distinguish between the two. Get up and walk around for 15 minutes to see if it's your body or your mind. Yes, just 15 minutes can tell you what's happening and how to respond. If it's your mind, give yourself a few hours of rest, then force yourself out of bed. If you're working, rest in your car or anywhere that gives you space and time to regroup. You don't need to explain yourself to friends/co-workers – whoever -- if you just need space. Just do it.

One of the things that I have found most helpful with myself, my patients, and private practice clients, is to delve into something inspiring. I find movies or books in which an individual or a group of people conquer insurmountable challenges, such as having been given horrific prognosis, yet prove them wrong, made it through imprisonment, fought for what they believed in, survived seemingly hopeless situations, gives me strength. Stepping out of one's own situation to view the success of an unconquerable will is inspirational.

SURVIVORS GUILT

I remember having serious survivor's guilt when my best friend died a week before her 41st birthday, shortly after I lost a 15-year-old friend to Cystic Fibrosis. I could not imagine why I was still living. I felt guilty having fun. I created a distance between my husband and me. I didn't want to laugh or be happy.

One night, I had a dream. In the dream, my best friend and I were on a road trip. She was lecturing me. She was telling me that it was my duty, my responsibility to enjoy life now. She told me I had a mission and that I had to keep going. To this day, I don't completely understand the dream, but it worked. I started to live again, understanding there must be a reason I'm still here. There's a reason that you are still here, even if you don't know what it is just yet. Grab on to it. Be grateful. Say, "Thank you," and embrace each moment.

TOOLS TO LIVE

Have a mini breakdown…get away from every one or just get with a good friend. If you have a spouse, you need to redefine your relationship and make sure that he/she has a support system. If you don't redefine the relationship, you may find yourself in it alone or at least feeling alone. People feel helpless when they cannot fix things, so they need specific things they can do. You need to set up clear ways your partner can help you. He/she cannot read your mind and may not be a natural nurturer or giver. Don't get mad, get clear. "I would like you to do the grocery shopping for me, please. This is what I need." "I would like you to give our daughter a bath at 7:00, as I'll be sick/tired." Be clear that your body has changed. It's ok to ask for help. Hire help if you can afford it. Let the house get messy. Use your energy to do fun things. Encourage your spouse to talk to someone if he/she cannot talk to you. Tell them that you love them, appreciate them and when you get well, you are going to travel the world together. Fake it if you have to…it helps. Set boundaries with your children and make sure that you and your partner are on the same page with them. Do not let the kids manipulate you because you feel guilty; they don't know they are hurting you. Love and be clear with them, "If you let mommy rest, we can do something special." Be proactive or you will not be able to continue at the pace you are going.

CHAPTER 14
THE LONG AND WINDING ROAD
TO RECOVERY

🚲 🚲 🚲

The entrance to the road to recovery is where we left off in book one. What I can say about it so far, is that it's a tricky one. On the one hand, you are ready (and so deserve) to celebrate. You're going to want to eat all of your favorite foods again, and possibly experience some new ones. It becomes very easy to take on a, "why not?" attitude when presented with decadence. Why not have two brownies, or a third glass of wine, or the family size, ice cream cake?

Or, maybe you'll gravitate toward extreme adventures like; hiking the Himalayas, or great white shark encounters of the third kind. Whatever your deal, just keep the mantra, "Steady as she goes." in the forefront of your mind. Depending on how long you were exposed to it, it could take your body years to fully recover from chemo. Even then, you may never fully recover. In some cases, the damage may be permanent, so go easy. By all means, enjoy, but don't go crazy, and set yourself back even further.

Remember this, if nothing; A compromised immune system puts you at risk of relapse. After all that treatment, your immune system is definitely compromised, so focus on detoxing your body first, and getting it into a healthy place that can withstand all the madcap adventures you've been looking forward to.

Once that soaks in, add this; remission has no guarantee of lasting forever. Even though cancer is heading into the "chronic" phase in the disease's life span, there is no actual cure for cancer, yet. It can come back, or your body could develop another type. In my family, there is a history of; breast, colon, endometrial, and pancreatic cancer (to name a few), so it would just be silly of me to think I could only get one, and I'm currently in my third remission, so I'm pretty sure I won't blindly assume I'm ever in the clear for good.

I don't care what "they" say. Even if you're in remission for over five years, do NOT think for a minute you get to just ride off into the sunset (cut and scene). For the rest of your life you must keep a balance between, "getting on with life," and "keeping an eye on it.". Get screened on a regular basis. How regular, should be decided between you and your doc, but if they say "no need," politely disagree. Too many fell for that romantic ideal, stopped screening, the cancer came back (or a new one developed), and it wasn't caught until it was late stage. I can tell you that I will never let more than a year go by before the next screening.

I keep picturing a recent moment, when I was sitting in the chemo chair, and a gal came bounding into the center. Elated, is the best word to describe her. She was dropping off a "thank you" lunch for the nurses, and posing for pics with them. You could tell, it was obvious, she was not only just in remission, but thought she was finally free of cancer, and all the goes with it, for good. I had that same feeling during my first remission. I'm sure, so did the journalist who had just lost her battle. I wanted to reach out and warn her, but how do you say, "Whoa, don't get too excited or comfortable there chica. This could just be a temporary reprieve." No one wants to be the wet blanket, but no one who's been there (and back), wants to see someone else blindsided by delusions of normality.

Once you've boosted your immune system back up to healthy levels, take time to invest in your dreams. I have a bucket list that grows almost daily, and I get such a thrill whenever one of them is about to be realized. My heart starts racing (in a good way) just thinking about it~ The biggest challenge, of course, is coming up with the funding for all these amazing experiences we plan, but we're no strangers to challenge now, are we.

Someone recently asked me who inspires me to keep fighting. Well, that's a long list, but the two people that came to mind immediately (that we all might know) were Dwayne, aka *The Rock,* Johnson and Ricky Gervais. Quite a pair I know, but here's why: The Rock is a fighter, and he doesn't let excuses come into play. "Be the hardest working person in the room." That's what I take from him. Ricky, is all about humor, and doing what you love. My favorite saying of his, "Don't let anyone tell you you're not good enough."

I remember, years back, someone I looked up to discouraged me from trying to record a CD of my music, stating it was far more work and expense than I understood, and that four months wasn't nearly enough time to get it done, but four months later I was sitting in my parents' kitchen, singing for my dad, while he stared down at the professionally recorded CD my friends and I made for him, for his 80th birthday. It's that type of mentality you need to bring to the cancer table. Don't let anyone convince you that you can't. Unless, of course, it's "You can't possibly eat that four gallon tub of ice cream and not gain a pound." Some things are simple logic peeps, to even the worst chemo brain.

I know, I already said this, but after three goes myself, I can't urge strongly enough to mentally prepare yourself for the cancer coming back. It could, even if you go; vegan, gluten free, take mega vitamins, and become a yoga master, so don't forget to balance awareness, with living it up. You need to build up a reserve of strength, for a possible second battle (or more). Don't wait too long to start doing those things you were looking forward to doing after you were done with chemo. Doing all those amazing things on my list, like; singing at The Festa Del Pesce in Italy, or walking along the Cliffs of Moher in Ireland, helped me to face another round, in ways I can hardly express.

Put rebuilding your immune system at the forefront. Eat healthier. Exercise more. Focus on replenishing all the good stuff your body had lost; glutamine, protein, vitamins, minerals, digestive enzymes and probiotics. Will it make a difference in long term remission? Who knows for sure, but you'll definitely feel healthier and physically stronger. That's a great place to be, if/when you do have to go back into battle.

There is one thing I discovered just before this book went to print. If you've been at it for a while, your body may have picked up the physical memory of being in fight mode (tension, hibernation, hanging onto chemo weight, etc.). Like a soldier home from active duty, you may need a little help transitioning back into (cancer is no longer at the center of my) life. Look for someone with Reiki skills and/or acupuncture or Qi Gong. There are lots of options, and with your new outlook on life you should be open to trying them. I did, and I'm amazed at the difference it makes.

Right, and with that my friend, I say get on with it. If you've read and followed through on everything to this point, then you should be feeling pretty powerful and calm. No matter where you are when you read this (treatment/remission), get on it. Get on with life, and squeeze every ounce of goodness from each day.

While you're doing that, I'm going to just pop over around the corner and have a quick chat with your loved ones...

CHAPTER 15
LETTER TO THE LOVED ONES (AND AN OUNCE OF PREVENTION)

🚲 🚲 🚲

I know, this is hard on you too. You wish you could blink and make their cancer go away. You're shocked at the realization, that they may leave this world. You want to help, but you know there's such a fine line between helpful and overbearing. What can you do? How can you be most helpful? First, and foremost, is to remain calm. If you're freaked out, then it'll stress them out, and stress does NOT do a body good. I'll give you some insights into how they are feeling, how you can help, and when we're done here, you can go to the website, where you'll find my top 12 list of useful gifts, so you can put a bow on that bounty of helpfulness.

Here's what I can tell you about most cancer patients:

TIRED

Some days and moments in a day, they'll be too tired to cook, clean, keep up with the mail, or have conversations with anyone. Bringing them frozen meals is nice, but fresh is better, since the microwave kills a lot of the nutrients in food. Think foods that are; easy to digest, high in protein and spicy. Everything smells and tastes weird to cancer patients, so avoid their favorite foods or you'll risk being the friend associated with them hating those foods forever.

SICK

Sometimes, it feels like a combination of the flu, morning sickness, and like their body is bruised from the inside out, and it comes and goes. They can feel relatively good one minute and turn grey the next. There are days they may be too sick to get themselves to chemo treatment/hospital and back, so offers for rides are great.

CRANKY

Thanks to a combination of life upheaval and steroids, they're going to have a significantly reduced tolerance for BS, so don't be surprised if they bite someone's head off for whining about a mutual friend's backhanded compliments, or whatever they'd normally go on for hours about in lively debate. On other days though, they'll crave to hear it all, just for the distraction. And then, there are those moments when they blurt out something uncharacteristically rude or socially unacceptable... Be patient with your semi tri-polar buddy.

VULNERABLE

Their immune systems are compromised, so stay away if you have even the slightest cold. Passing that on, could land them in the hospital. This is no joke. Also, if you bring them any raw foods make sure they get washed with antibacterial cleanser. Raw fish/meat and grapefruit (for most) are off-limits until their doctor says so. Because they're so vulnerable, the best place for them is home most of the time, so going out to bars or gyms or traveling of any kind while they're in treatment is mostly off limits. They need to stay as protected as possible. However, they also need fresh air, so short walks (as long as they're protected from the sun) or bike rides will do them good. Remember, they are the ones that are vulnerable to germs, so when you're out and about with them, be the one who opens the door, presses the elevator button, and carry anti-bacterial wipes or gel in case they forgot to carry theirs.

PROUD

They may be too proud to tell you when they need something. Sometimes, you may have to discreetly investigate to find out their needs and fill them, if you can. It's also very important you share that list of needs with others. Your friend-in-need would never want to see you collapse from the weight of struggle to help them. It's also extremely important to set aside any differences with mutual friends/family. Conflicts only deplete what little energy they have.

SAD

Even if they go on antidepressants, they will have sad moments. Let them have 'em, but don't let them feel sorry for themselves for too long. How long, is up to you two to decide. Some people need a minute, some need a day. Remember, the power of endorphins, so offer up their favorite distraction whenever it's suitable..

CONFUSED

Chemo brain is kind of like being stoned. Your otherwise bright friend will forget what he or she was saying mid-sentence, where keys were left, and (sigh) much, much more. Be kind and don't expect them to remember much of anything. Don't be offended if they forget plans, or even put the wrong date and time in their calendar. There is no telling how long this will last after treatment is finished. On that note, dealing with bills and paperwork (soooo much paperwork), can be really confusing, even without chemo brain. So, if you're a whiz with numbers, and navigating through bureaucratic BS, then by all means, raise your hand for this assignment. That is a much appreciated skill.

UNATTRACTIVE

This is worse for some, more than others, but no one will feel like an amazing and alluring person. Cancer patients are going through a serious arse whooping and it'll show. There is nothing sexy about cancer. They could really benefit from a little TLC, so if you have the means to provide anything like; hair treatments, wigs, new hats, massages or facials, these are the gifts that make a difference. One of my most appreciated gifts was a trip to the local day spa, for an herbal detox wrap at the end of a chemo cycle. It felt good to be pampered, and I was surprised how much faster I bounced back from the latest cycle. Just remember, keep it to super clean environments for safety's sake. If you're not sure, just call the cancer treatment center and they'll let you know.

SLIGHTLY DELUDED

They'll have days when they're feeling great, and want to take it all on themselves. Knowing when to jump in, and smack some sense into them is an acquired skill. Flying home that Thanksgiving probably should have been one of those times, but even more so, was when I decided to take the coaster train from the airport back home. This involved bus rides and lugging stuff quite a ways. One of my equally obstinate friends, got a hold of me shortly after landing and commanded I sit still, and let her drive down to pick me up. This is the hard part. People who are sick, don't mean to question you, per se. They just have those moments where they travel a little too far into denial city, and they need a little nudge back in the right direction.

The most important thing you can do, is to NOT treat your friend like a dying person. Instead, carry on like they are just going through a rough patch, need some distraction and TLC, like with a bad breakup, "That c punk is a loser. You're better off without 'em." Yeah, something like that. Your friend doesn't want to talk about cancer 24/7 and gets enough of that, as it is. Don't try to control or nag either. They have very little control over their body or life right now, so sometimes he or she will want to exert the right to have a drink, or go shopping. If they aren't keeling over, then let 'em have that moment of normalcy.

Now that we've covered what you can do for them, let's get to the business of what you need to do for yourself. Take this opportunity to ask yourself what you would do if the tables were turned, you were diagnosed with cancer, and had to go through treatment. Do you have a written and witnessed will? Do you have long term disability insurance? Do you have life insurance? Do you have health insurance? The answer to all of the above should be a resounding, "YES." No, I didn't pick up a new career as an insurance salesman. I am living proof that when the shite hits the fan, these insurance policies will save your bacon.

I've thanked Ian many times (at least in my head, and to others), the guy who convinced me to sign up for long term disability insurance when I was hired on at my last job. I balked at it because, "I'm healthy as a horse." I said. "I'm rarely ever sick." Well, duh. It's not something you sign up for when you're sick. Having it isn't a sign of weakness. Insurance is something you'll be oh so grateful for if/when the moment hits.

When you sign up for these insurance plans, do NOT go for the cheapest option (unless it's the best). A good friend's husband was going to lower his life insurance premium to save them a few hundred a year. Not two months later (I kid you not), he died, suddenly. It was a shock to us all. He was a relatively healthy guy. If he had gone through with cutting back on his life insurance, his wife and kids would've been okay for a year or so, but then, they would've had to start making sacrifices. As it stands, his kids will all have the opportunity to complete college and his wife can stay put in their home for as long as she lives. She would trade all of that to have him back, there is no doubt, but it's very comforting to know that he chose an option that would continue to provide for his family for a good many years to come .

Don't think you need long term disability insurance? 1 in 2 people will face cancer in their lifetime. Those are real statistics. Go look 'em up. You really think you can beat those odds? And that's just cancer. You could fall off a ladder, get hit by an uninsured driver, or run into a tree while downhill skiing...you are not immune.

Do a good amount of research on long term disability plans

before buying anything, and remember this; these people may be friendly, but they are NOT your friends. For many, their sole purpose is to try and find any loophole to get out of paying any funds out when a disability claim is made.

For example, I have this friend who took whatever was offered to them without doing any research or comparisons of what's out there, and the people she spoke to at this particular disability insurance company, were always pleasant, professional, and seemed genuinely sympathetic to her plight.

However, while she was basking in the glow of their warm fuzzies, the company hired someone to cyber stalk her, to dig up whatever so-called evidence they could find, to avoid approving long term disability coverage. How does she know? The jerk actually called her doc and said (with a suspicious tone), "We have a file 'this thick' on her...did you know she goes swimming, goes for walks on the beach and plays guitar?" "Eh, yes." was the reply. "These are all therapeutic, and what someone should do in a genuine attempt to recover."

That was over a year ago, but the claim is still unsettled, in limbo. You would think a diagnosis of Stage IV cancer would be enough to stamp the file and move on to the next, but it isn't, so be aware now, that when it comes to these plans, you get what you pay for, and no matter how much you pay, you must be prepared to fight for what's right. I know, like anyone dealing with a life threatening illness needs that kind of stress, but this is the reality of it. Before all of this I was a hopelessly romantic *optimista*. Now...I'm more of a hopeful *realista*.

Whatever you take away from this book, I hope it is that; life is as good as you make it. It's meant to be lived NOW, not in a few years, after you've saved up enough vacation time money, are in remission or lost that extra weight. Now, fer fkssake. Invest in those safety nets, in case the shite hits the fan, be preemptive, and get screened before symptoms could possibly arise. Then, go live the life that makes you genuinely happy. Forgive and forget the jerks. Live and let live. Love and be loveable. Contribute to society once in a while, and be kind to those around you, because you never know when you're going to need them for a ride to your next colonoscopy or PET scan~

Remember, this book is meant to be a quick and to-the-point reference guide. You'll find plenty more information on the website: www.theccardandme.com. And if you found this guide to be useful, please help to spread the word. Talk about it at work, post on your social media, like *The C Card and Me* Facebook page, and take a moment to review it online.

Imagine if after you first discover you have cancer you are bombarded with stories of real people, just like you and me, who are actually beating it. Ooooh I think we're on to something...

EPILOGUE

🚲 🚲 🚲

Writing these guides has been epiphanetic (yup, I just made up that one) for me. I'll admit, I've been trying to run away from a life with cancer since the day I was diagnosed; hiding from site when I'm on chemo and calling it, "going to work," (confusing the hell out of anyone who knew I was on disability). And trying to maintain the lifestyle I was accustomed to (pre-cancer), was often an exercise in disaster.

The thing is, I love to feel useful. I have an inherent need to feel useful. Being disabled and on debilitating cancer treatments has not made me feel useful. I kept dreaming of "getting my body back" and my old way of life, working 24/7 and being an oh so busy, professional geek with the office, the salary and the perks (and the stresses) that go with it.

Over the past few years, when people I meet, ask me what I do for a living, I'd kind of freeze, not sure what to say..."I used to be an IT Director." That would usually be my response. I would often avoid the cancer topic, because I didn't want to be that person...you know, the one who always brings the party down a notch with their tragic story.

The thing is (and pay attention, this is the epiphanetic moment), once you face cancer, it is and will always be a part of you. There is no going back to the exact life you had before it, and why the fek would you? There is something about your former life that allowed this cancer to invade your body and your world. Never lose sight of that.

The treatments will humble you, age you and the longer you are on them, the greater the chances of permanent damage. Once you get that into your thick skull, then you will see the grand opportunity you have to redefine yourself, your world.

I have been hitting my head against that proverbial brick

wall, trying to get my brain to work like an IT Director again because that's what it has known for decades now and when I felt most useful, but you know what they say about heads and brick walls…

One fascinating thing about the effects of chemo brain is that it puts you into a singular line of thinking. The past is fuzzy, the future is hazy (at best), but what is right in front of you is clear as a bell. What could be more useful than being the living proof you can still have a great life after being diagnosed with late stage cancer? And how about the next best thing…because you read this guide and took heed, you not only caught your cancer early enough to nip it in the bud with the briefest of treatments, but you were well insured and didn't have to worry about losing your home, your car, or your dreams of the future? How cool would that be? Right, then. Time for the re-definition of Ali (I'll go first, you follow).

"Hi, my name is Ali Gilmore. What do I do? I'm a writer and a public speaker. What do I write and speak about? I make people less afraid of cancer and better prepared to face it. Yes, yes it is a cool job. It's very rewarding and it makes me feel incredibly useful~"

HONOR PAGE
A special recognition to some of the fighters in my friends' lives

🚲 🚲 🚲

Amanda Downing Bahr for Robert Michael Downing of
Fallbrook, CA

Ana Couch for Kristin Coriano of San Diego, CA

Bernadette O'Neill for Jennifer O'Halloran and Nora O'Neill of
Youghal, Ireland

Christina Boles-Medeima for Cindy Lu James of Everett, WA

Debalou Riebe for Karolyn Cavanaugh-Blank of Everett, WA

Dianne Pollock for Jack Breheny of Belfast, Ireland

The Giblin Family for Sean Giblin of Galway, Ireland

Hal Gilmore for Alice Gilmore of Detroit, MI

Ilene Robbins for Elsie Robbins of Corona, CA

Jen Conrads for Victoria Swankie of Woodland Hills, CA

Lawrence & Shannon Kahn for Susan Kahn, Jeffrey Beada and
Gary Kahn of Hillside, NJ

Lisa Dujat for Kymmie Bisnett of Syracuse, NY

Margaret Lum for Frank Lum of Honolulu, HI

Pete Davidson for Joan Davidson of New York, NY

Rick and Michelle Nelson for Lorna E. Nelson of Ballard, WA

Stewart Valenzuela for Ron, aka Hobbit, Valenzuela of Maui, HI

Tawnya Friend-Jackson for Pat Friend of Everett, WA

ABOUT THE AUTHOR

🚲 🚲 🚲

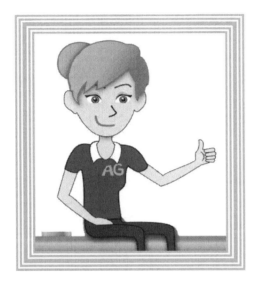

Ali Gilmore was born in Seattle, Washington. She is the youngest of seven and the daughter of a Stage III cancer survivor. Since her late stage diagnosis in 2010, Ali has been striving to live life to the fullest and to reach her lifetime achievement goal of making over a million people less afraid of cancer and better prepared to face it, through *The C Card and Me* books and motivational speaking engagements.

When she isn't photographing MLS players or traveling the world, tackling the items on her ever growing bucket list, Ali is at home in Oceanside, California, pursuing creative endeavors and enjoying the beach town life. Read more about Ali and her ever growing bucket list at: www.aligilmore.com.

To book Ali for a memorable speaking engagement, contact: michelle@shinepretc.com. Be inspired.

Made in the USA
San Bernardino, CA
07 April 2016